DRUG ADDICTION

SCIENCE AND TREATMENT

PUBLIC HEALTH IN THE 21ST CENTURY

Additional books in this series can be found on Nova's website
under the Series tab.

Additional E-books in this series can be found on Nova's website
under the E-book tab.

ALCOHOL AND DRUG ABUSE

Additional books in this series can be found on Nova's website
under the Series tab.

Additional E-books in this series can be found on Nova's website
under the E-book tab.

PUBLIC HEALTH IN THE 21ST CENTURY

DRUG ADDICTION

SCIENCE AND TREATMENT

NATHAN JACOBS

AND

LAURA C. DUBOIS

EDITORS

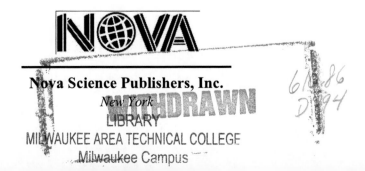

Nova Science Publishers, Inc.

New York

Copyright © 2012 by Nova Science Publishers, Inc.

For permission to use material from this book please contact us:
Telephone 631-231-7269; Fax 631-231-8175
Web Site: http://www.novapublishers.com

Additional color graphics may be available in the e-book version of this book.

Library of Congress Cataloging-in-Publication Data

ISBN 978-1-61470-004-3

Published by Nova Science Publishers, Inc. † *New York*

CONTENTS

PREFACE

This book provides scientific information about the disease of drug addiction, including the many harmful consequences of drug abuse and the basic approaches that have been developed to prevent and treat the disease.

Chapter 1- Throughout much of the last century, scientists studying drug abuse labored in the shadows of powerful myths and misconceptions about the nature of addiction. When science began to study addictive behavior in the 1930s, people addicted to drugs were thought to be morally flawed and lacking in willpower. Those views shaped society's responses to drug abuse, treating it as a moral failing rather than a health problem, which led to an emphasis on punitive rather than preventative and therapeutic actions. Today, thanks to science, our views and our responses to drug abuse have changed dramatically. Groundbreaking discoveries about the brain have revolutionized our understanding of drug addiction, enabling us to respond effectively to the problem.

Chapter 2- Drug addiction is a complex illness. It is characterized by intense and, at times, uncontrollable drug craving, along with compulsive drug seeking and use that persists even in the face of devastating consequences.

Many people do not realize that addiction is a brain disease. While the path to drug addiction begins with the act of taking drugs, over time a person's ability to choose not to do so becomes compromised, and seeking and consuming the drug becomes compulsive. This behavior results largely from the effects of prolonged drug exposure on brain functioning. Addiction affects multiple brain circuits, including those involved in reward and motivation, learning and memory, and inhibitory control over behavior. Some individuals are more vulnerable than others to becoming addicted, depending on genetic makeup, age of exposure to drugs, other environmental influences, and the interplay of all these factors.

Chapter 3- Drug addiction has well-recognized cognitive, behavioral, and physiological characteristics that contribute to continued use of drugs despite the harmful consequences. Scientists have also found that chronic drug abuse alters the brain's anatomy and chemistry and that these changes can last for months or years after the individual has stopped using drugs. This transformation may help explain why addicts are at a high risk of relapse to drug abuse even after long periods of abstinence and why they persist in seeking drugs despite deleterious consequences.

In: Drug Addiction: Science and Treatment   ISBN: 978-1-61470-004-3
Editors: N. Jacobs and L. C. Dubois   © 2012 Nova Science Publishers, Inc.

Chapter 1

DRUGS, BRAINS AND BEHAVIOR: THE SCIENCE OF ADDICTION*

National Institute on Drug Abuse

"Drug addiction is a brain disease that can be treated."

Nora D. Volkow, M.D.
Director, National Institute
on Drug Abuse

PREFACE

How Science Has Revolutionized the Understanding of Drug Addiction

Throughout much of the last century, scientists studying drug abuse labored in the shadows of powerful myths and misconceptions about the nature of addiction. When science began to study addictive behavior in the 1930s, people addicted to drugs were thought to be morally flawed and lacking in willpower. Those views shaped society's responses to drug

---

* This is an edited, reformatted and augmented version of a National Institute on Drug Abuse publication, dated April 2007, Revised February 2008, Revised August 2010.

abuse, treating it as a moral failing rather than a health problem, which led to an emphasis on punitive rather than preventative and therapeutic actions. Today, thanks to science, our views and our responses to drug abuse have changed dramatically. Groundbreaking discoveries about the brain have revolutionized our understanding of drug addiction, enabling us to respond effectively to the problem.

As a result of scientific research, we know that addiction is a disease that affects both brain and behavior. We have identified many of the biological and environmental factors and are beginning to search for the genetic variations that contribute to the development and progression of the disease. Scientists use this knowledge to develop effective prevention and treatment approaches that reduce the toll drug abuse takes on individuals, families, and communities.

Despite these advances, many people today do not understand why individuals become addicted to drugs or how drugs change the brain to foster compulsive drug abuse. This booklet aims to fill that knowledge gap by providing scientific information about the disease of drug addiction, including the many harmful consequences of drug abuse and the basic approaches that have been developed to prevent and treat the disease. At the National Institute on Drug Abuse (NIDA), we believe that increased understanding of the basics of addiction will empower people to make informed choices in their own lives, adopt science-based policies and programs that reduce drug abuse and addiction in their communities, and support scientific research that improves the Nation's well-being.

Nora D. Volkow, M.D
Director
National Institute on Drug Abuse

INTRODUCTION

Why Study Drug Abuse and Addiction?

Abuse and addiction to alcohol, nicotine, and illegal substances cost Americans upwards of half a trillion dollars a year, considering their combined medical, economic, criminal, and social impact. Every year, abuse of illicit drugs and alcohol contributes to the death of more than 100,000 Americans, while tobacco is linked to an estimated 440,000 deaths per year. *People of all ages suffer the harmful consequences of drug abuse and addiction.*

- *Babies* exposed to legal and illegal drugs in the womb may be born premature and underweight. This drug exposure can slow the child's intellectual development and affect behavior later in life.
- *Adolescents* who abuse drugs often act out, do poorly academically, and drop out of school. They are at risk of unplanned pregnancies, violence, and infectious diseases.
- *Adults* who abuse drugs often have problems thinking clearly, remembering, and paying attention. They often develop poor social behaviors as a result of their drug abuse, and their work performance and personal relationships suffer.
- *Parents'* drug abuse often means chaotic, stress-filled homes and child abuse and neglect. Such conditions harm the well-being and development of children in the home and may set the stage for drug abuse in the next generation.

How Does Science Provide Solutions for Drug Abuse and Addiction?

Scientists study the effects that drugs have on the brain and on people's behavior. They use this information to develop programs for preventing drug abuse and for helping people recover from addiction. Further research helps transfer these ideas into practice in our communities.

I. DRUG ABUSE AND ADDICTION

What Is Drug Addiction?

Addiction is defined as a chronic, relapsing brain disease that is characterized by compulsive drug seeking and use, despite harmful consequences. It is considered a brain disease because drugs change the brain—they change its structure and how it works. These brain changes can be long lasting, and can lead to the harmful behaviors seen in people who abuse drugs.

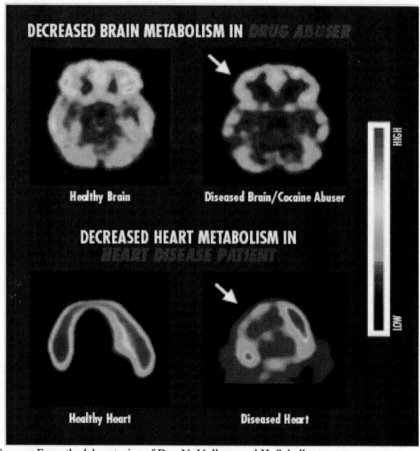

Source: From the laboratories of Drs. N. Volkow and H. Schelbert.

Addiction is similar to other diseases, such as heart disease. Both disrupt the normal, healthy functioning of the underlying organ, have serious harmful consequences, are preventable, treatable, and if left untreated, can last a lifetime.

Why Do People Take Drugs?

In general, people begin taking drugs for a variety of reasons:

- *To feel good.* Most abused drugs produce intense feelings of pleasure. This initial sensation of euphoria is followed by other effects, which differ with the type of drug used. For example, with stimulants such as cocaine, the "high" is followed by feelings of power, self-confidence, and increased energy. In contrast, the euphoria caused by opiates such as heroin is followed by feelings of relaxation and satisfaction.

- *To feel better.* Some people who suffer from social anxiety, stress-related disorders, and depression begin abusing drugs in an attempt to lessen feelings of distress. Stress can play a major role in beginning drug use, continuing drug abuse, or relapse in patients recovering from addiction.

- *To do better.* The increasing pressure that some individuals feel to chemically enhance or improve their athletic or cognitive performance can similarly play a role in initial experimentation and continued drug abuse.

- *Curiosity and "because others are doing it."* In this respect adolescents are particularly vulnerable because of the strong influence of peer pressure; they are more likely, for example, to engage in "thrilling" and "daring" behaviors.

If Taking Drugs Makes People Feel Good or Better, What's the Problem?

At first, people may perceive what seem to be positive effects with drug use. They also may believe that they can control their use; however, drugs can quickly take over their lives. Consider how a social drinker can become intoxicated, put himself behind a wheel and quickly turn a pleasurable activity into a tragedy for him and others. Over time, if drug use continues, pleasurable activities become less pleasurable, and drug abuse becomes necessary for abusers to simply feel "normal." Drug abusers reach a point where they seek and take drugs, despite the tremendous problems caused for themselves and their loved ones. Some individuals may start to feel the need to take higher or more frequent doses, even in the early stages of their drug use.

Is Continued Drug Abuse a Voluntary Behavior?

The initial decision to take drugs is mostly voluntary. However, when drug abuse takes over, a person's ability to exert self control can become seriously impaired.

Examples of Risk and Protective Factors		
Risk Factors	Domain	Protective Factors
Early Aggressive Behavior	Individual	Self-Control
Poor Social Skills	Individual	Positive Relationships
Lack of Parental Supervision	Family	Parental Monitoring and Support
Substance Abuse	Peer	Academic Competence
Drug Availability	School	Anti-Drug Use Policies
Poverty	Community	Strong Neighborhood Attachment

Brain imaging studies from drug-addicted individuals show physical changes in areas of the brain that are critical to judgment, decisionmaking, learning and memory, and behavior control. Scientists believe that these changes alter the way the brain works, and may help explain the compulsive and destructive behaviors of addiction.

Why Do Some People Become Addicted to Drugs, While Others Do Not?

As with any other disease, vulnerability to addiction differs from person to person. In general, the more risk factors an individual has, the greater the chance that taking drugs will lead to abuse and addiction. "Protective" factors reduce a person's risk of developing addiction.

What Factors Determine if a Person Will Become Addicted?

No single factor determines whether a person will become addicted to drugs. The overall risk for addiction is impacted by the biological makeup of the individual—it can even be influenced by gender or ethnicity, his or her developmental stage, and the surrounding social environment (e.g., conditions at home, at school, and in the neighborhood).

Which Biological Factors Increase Risk of Addiction?

Scientists estimate that genetic factors account for between 40 and 60 percent of a person's vulnerability to addiction, including the effects of environment on gene expression and function. Adolescents and individuals with mental disorders are at greater risk of drug abuse and addiction than the general population.

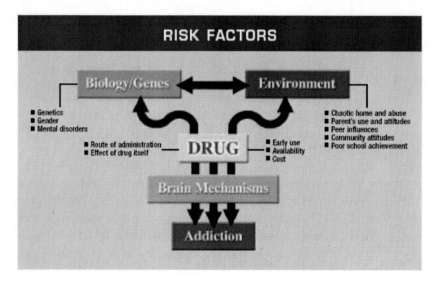

What Environmental Factors Increase the Risk of Addiction?

- *Home and Family.* The influence of the home environment is usually most important in childhood. Parents or older family members who abuse alcohol or drugs or who engage in criminal behavior can increase children's risks of developing their own drug problems.
- *Peer and School.* Friends and acquaintances have the greatest influence during adolescence. Drug-abusing peers can sway even those without risk factors to try drugs for the first time. Academic failure or poor social skills can put a child further at risk for drug abuse.

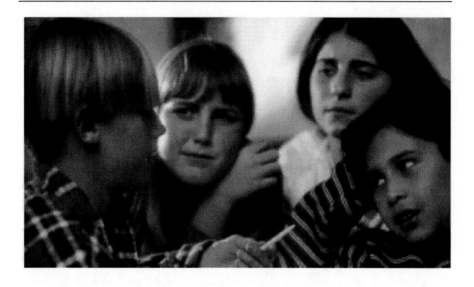

What other Factors Increase the Risk of Addiction?

- *Early Use.* Although taking drugs at any age can lead to addiction, research shows that the earlier a person begins to use drugs the more likely they are to progress to more serious abuse. This may reflect the harmful effect that drugs can have on the developing brain; it also may result from a constellation of early biological and social vulnerability factors, including genetic susceptibility, mental illness, unstable family relationships, and exposure to physical or sexual abuse. Still, the fact remains that early use is a strong indicator of problems ahead, among them, substance abuse and addiction.

- *Method of Administration.* Smoking a drug or injecting it into a vein increases its addictive potential. Both smoked and injected drugs enter the brain within seconds, producing a powerful rush of pleasure. However, this intense "high" can fade within a few minutes, taking the abuser down to lower, more normal levels. It is a starkly felt contrast, and scientists believe that this low feeling drives individuals to repeated drug abuse in an attempt to recapture the high pleasurable state.

The Brain Continues to Develop into Adulthood and Undergoes Dramatic Changes During Adolescence

One of the brain areas still maturing during adolescence is the prefrontal cortex—the part of the brain that enables us to assess situations, make sound decisions, and keep our emotions and desires under control. The fact that this critical part of an adolescent's brain is still a work-in-progress puts them at increased risk for poor decisions (such as trying drugs or continued abuse). Also, introducing drugs while the brain is still developing may have profound and long-lasting consequences.

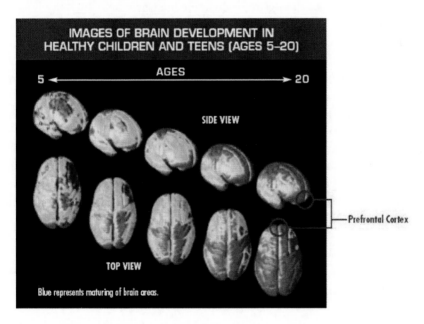

IMAGES OF BRAIN DEVELOPMENT IN HEALTHY CHILDREN AND TEENS (AGES 5–20)

AGES

5 ⟵————————————————⟶ 20

SIDE VIEW

Prefrontal Cortex

TOP VIEW

Blue represents maturing of brain areas.

II. PREVENTING DRUG ABUSE: THE BEST STRATEGY

Why is Adolescence a Critical Time for Preventing Drug Addiction?

As noted previously, early use of drugs increases a person's chances of more serious drug abuse and addiction. Remember, drugs change brains—and this can lead to addiction and other serious problems. So preventing early use of drugs or alcohol may reduce the risk of progressing to later abuse and addiction. Risk of drug abuse increases greatly during times of transition, such as changing schools, moving, or divorce. If we can prevent drug abuse, we can prevent drug addiction. In early adolescence, when children advance from elementary through middle school, they face new and challenging social and academic situations. Often during this period, children are exposed to abusable substances such as cigarettes and alcohol for the first time. When they enter high school, teens may encounter greater availability of drugs, drug abuse by older teens, and social activities where drugs are used.

At the same time, many behaviors that are a normal aspect of their development, such as the desire to do something new or risky, may increase teen tendencies to experiment with drugs. Some teens may give in to the urging of drug-abusing friends to share the experience with them. Others may think that taking drugs (such as steroids) will improve their appearance or their athletic performance or that abusing substances such as alcohol or ecstasy (MDMA) will ease their anxiety in social situations.

Teens' still-developing judgment and decisionmaking skills may limit their ability to assess risks accurately and make sound decisions about using drugs. Drug and alcohol abuse can disrupt brain function in areas critical to motivation, memory, learning, judgment, and behavior control. So, it is not surprising that teens who abuse alcohol and other drugs often have family and school problems, poor academic performance, health-related problems (including mental health), and involvement with the juvenile justice system.

Can Science-Validated Programs Prevent Drug Addiction in Youth?

Yes. The term "science-validated" means that these programs have been rationally designed based on current knowledge, rigorously tested, and shown to produce positive results. Scientists have developed a broad range of programs that positively alter the balance between risk and protective factors for drug abuse in families, schools, and communities. Research has shown that science-validated programs, such as those described in NIDA's Preventing Drug Use among Children and Adolescents: A Research-Based Guide for Parents, Educators, and Community Leaders, can significantly reduce early use of tobacco, alcohol, and illicit drugs.

Drug abuse starts early and peaks in teen years

How Do Science-Validated Prevention Programs Work?

These prevention programs work to boost protective factors and eliminate or reduce risk factors for drug use. The programs are designed for various ages and can be designed for individual or group settings, such as the school and home. There are three types of programs—

- *Universal programs* address risk and protective factors common to all children in a given setting, such as a school or community.
- *Selective programs* target groups of children and teens who have factors that further increase their risk of drug abuse.
- *Indicated programs* are designed for youth who have already begun abusing drugs.

Are All Prevention Programs Effective in Reducing Drug Abuse?

When science-validated substance abuse prevention programs are properly implemented by schools and communities, alcohol, tobacco, and illicit drug abuse are reduced. Such programs help teachers, parents, and healthcare professionals shape youths' perceptions about the risks of drug abuse. While many events and cultural factors affect drug abuse trends, when youths perceive drug abuse as harmful, they reduce their level of abuse.

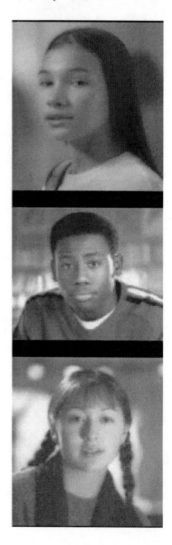

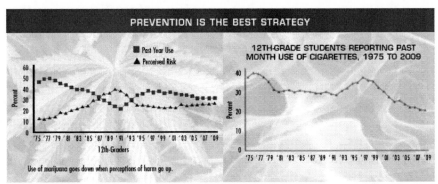

Source: 2009 Monitoring the Future survey. University of Michigan, with funding from the National Institute on Drug Abuse.

Good news: Cigarette smoking is at its lowest point since NIDA began tracking it in 1975. But declines in illicit drug use, especially marijuana, have stalled in the past few years. Prevention efforts should be redoubled to counter this troubling trend.

For more information on prevention, see NIDA's most recent edition of *Preventing Drug Use among Children and Adolescents: A Research-Based Guide for Parents, Educators, and Community Leaders,* at *www.drugabuse. gov/Prevention/Prevopen.html.*

III. Drugs and the Brain

Introducing the Human Brain

The human brain is the most complex organ in the body. This three-pound mass of gray and white matter sits at the center of all human activity—you need it to drive a car, to enjoy a meal, to breathe, to create an artistic masterpiece, and to enjoy everyday activities. In brief, the brain regulates your basic body functions; enables you to interpret and respond to everything you experience; and shapes your thoughts, emotions, and behavior.

The brain is made up of many parts that all work together as a team. Different parts of the brain are responsible for coordinating and performing specific functions. Drugs can alter important brain areas that are necessary for life-sustaining functions and can drive the compulsive drug abuse that marks addiction. Brain areas affected by drug abuse—

- *The brain stem* controls basic functions critical to life, such as heart rate, breathing, and sleeping.
- *The limbic system* contains the brain's reward circuit—it links together a number of brain structures that control and regulate our ability to feel pleasure. Feeling pleasure motivates us to repeat behaviors such as eating—actions that are critical to our existence. The limbic system is activated when we perform these activities— and also by drugs of abuse. In addition, the limbic system is responsible for our perception of other emotions, both positive and negative, which explains the mood-altering properties of many drugs.
- *The cerebral cortex* is divided into areas that control specific functions. Different areas process information from our senses, enabling us to see, feel, hear, and taste. The front part of the cortex, the frontal cortex or forebrain, is the thinking center of the brain; it powers our ability to think, plan, solve problems, and make decisions.

How Does the Brain Communicate?

The brain is a communications center consisting of billions of neurons, or nerve cells. Networks of neurons pass messages back and forth to different structures within the brain, the spinal column, and the peripheral nervous system. These nerve networks coordinate and regulate everything we feel, think, and do.

Neuron to Neuron
Each nerve cell in the brain sends and receives messages in the form of electrical impulses. Once a cell receives and processes a message, it sends it on to other neurons.

Neurotransmitters—The Brain's Chemical Messengers
The messages are carried between neurons by chemicals called neurotransmitters. (They transmit messages between neurons.)

Receptors—The Brain's Chemical Receivers
The neurotransmitter attaches to a specialized site on the receiving cell called a receptor. A neurotransmitter and its receptor operate like a "key and lock," an exquisitely specific mechanism that ensures that each receptor will

forward the appropriate message only after interacting with the right kind of neurotransmitter.

Transporters—The Brain's Chemical Recyclers

Located on the cell that releases the neurotransmitter, transporters recycle these neurotransmitters (i.e., bring them back into the cell that released them), thereby shutting off the signal between neurons.

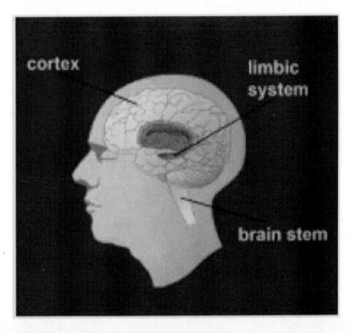

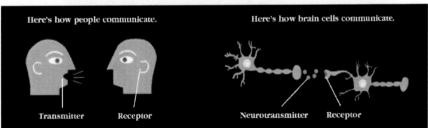

Concept courtesy: B.K. Madras.

To send a message a brain cell releases a chemical (neurotransmitter) into the space separating two cells called the synapse. The neurotransmitter crosses the synapse and attaches to proteins (receptors) on the receiving brain cell. This causes changes in the receiving brain cell and the message is delivered.

How Do Drugs Work in the Brain?

Drugs are chemicals. They work in the brain by tapping into the brain's communication system and interfering with the way nerve cells normally send, receive, and process information. Some drugs, such as marijuana and heroin, can activate neurons because their chemical structure mimics that of a natural neurotransmitter. This similarity in structure "fools" receptors and allows the drugs to lock onto and activate the nerve cells. Although these drugs mimic brain chemicals, they don't activate nerve cells in the same way as a natural neurotransmitter, and they lead to abnormal messages being transmitted through the network.

Other drugs, such as amphetamine or cocaine, can cause the nerve cells to release abnormally large amounts of natural neurotransmitters or prevent the normal recycling of these brain chemicals. This disruption produces a greatly amplified message, ultimately disrupting communication channels. The difference in effect can be described as the difference between someone whispering into your ear and someone shouting into a microphone.

How Do Drugs Work in the Brain to Produce Pleasure?

Most drugs of abuse directly or indirectly target the brain's reward system by flooding the circuit with dopamine. Dopamine is a neurotransmitter present in regions of the brain that regulate movement, emotion, cognition, motivation, and feelings of pleasure. The overstimulation of this system, which rewards our natural behaviors, produces the euphoric effects sought by people who abuse drugs and teaches them to repeat the behavior.

How Does Stimulation of the Brain's Pleasure Circuit Teach Us to Keep Taking Drugs?

Our brains are wired to ensure that we will repeat life-sustaining activities by associating those activities with pleasure or reward. Whenever this reward circuit is activated, the brain notes that something important is happening that needs to be remembered, and teaches us to do it again and again, without thinking about it. Because drugs of abuse stimulate the same circuit, we learn to abuse drugs in the same way.

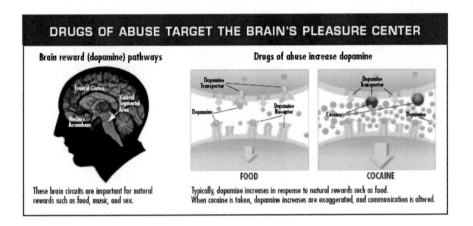

DRUGS OF ABUSE TARGET THE BRAIN'S PLEASURE CENTER

Brain reward (dopamine) pathways

Drugs of abuse increase dopamine

FOOD   COCAINE

These brain circuits are important for natural rewards such as food, music, and sex.

Typically, dopamine increases in response to natural rewards such as food. When cocaine is taken, dopamine increases are exaggerated, and communication is altered.

Why Are Drugs More Addictive than Natural Rewards?

When some drugs of abuse are taken, they can release 2 to 10 times the amount of dopamine that natural rewards do. In some cases, this occurs almost immediately (as when drugs are smoked or injected), and the effects can last much longer than those produced by natural rewards. The resulting effects on the brain's pleasure circuit dwarfs those produced by naturally rewarding behaviors such as eating and sex. The effect of such a powerful reward strongly motivates people to take drugs again and again. This is why scientists sometimes say that drug abuse is something we learn to do very, very well.

What Happens to Your Brain if You Keep Taking Drugs?

Just as we turn down the volume on a radio that is too loud, the brain adjusts to the overwhelming surges in dopamine (and other neurotransmitters) by producing less dopamine or by reducing the number of receptors that can receive signals. As a result, dopamine's impact on the reward circuit of a drug abuser's brain can become abnormally low, and the ability to experience any pleasure is reduced. This is why the abuser eventually feels flat, lifeless, and depressed, and is unable to enjoy things that previously brought them pleasure. Now, they need to take drugs just to try and bring their dopamine function back up to normal. And, they must take larger amounts of the drug than they first did to create the dopamine high—an effect known as tolerance.

How Does Long-Term Drug Taking Affect Brain Circuits?

We know that the same sort of mechanisms involved in the development of tolerance can eventually lead to profound changes in neurons and brain circuits, with the potential to severely compromise the long-term health of the brain. For example, glutamate is another neurotransmitter that influences the reward circuit and the ability to learn. When the optimal concentration of glutamate is altered by drug abuse, the brain attempts to compensate for this change, which can cause impairment in cognitive function. Similarly, long-term drug abuse can trigger adaptations in habit or nonconscious memory systems. Conditioning is one example of this type of learning, whereby environmental cues become associated with the drug experience and can trigger uncontrollable cravings if the individual is later exposed to these cues, even without the drug itself being available. This learned "reflex" is extremely robust and can emerge even after many years of abstinence.

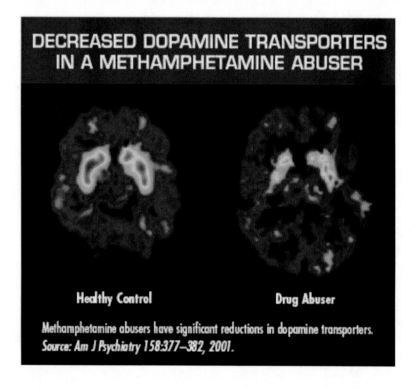

DECREASED DOPAMINE TRANSPORTERS IN A METHAMPHETAMINE ABUSER

Healthy Control   Drug Abuser

Methamphetamine abusers have significant reductions in dopamine transporters.
Source: Am J Psychiatry 158:377–382, 2001.

What other Brain Changes Occur with Abuse?

Chronic exposure to drugs of abuse disrupts the way critical brain structures interact to control and inhibit behaviors related to drug abuse. Just as continued abuse may lead to tolerance or the need for higher drug dosages to produce an effect, it may also lead to addiction, which can drive an abuser to seek out and take drugs compulsively. Drug addiction erodes a person's self-control and ability to make sound decisions, while sending intense impulses to take drugs.

For more information on drugs and the brain, order NIDA's Teaching Packets CD-ROM series or the Mind Over Matter series at www.drugabuse. gov/parent-teacher.html. These items and others are available to the public free of charge.

IV. ADDICTION AND HEALTH

What Are the Medical Consequences of Drug Addiction?

Individuals who suffer from addiction often have one or more accompanying medical issues, including lung and cardiovascular disease, stroke, cancer, and mental disorders. Imaging scans, chest X-rays, and blood tests show the damaging effects of drug abuse throughout the body. For example, tests show that tobacco smoke causes cancer of the mouth, throat, larynx, blood, lungs, stomach, pancreas, kidney, bladder, and cervix. In addition, some drugs of abuse, such as inhalants, are toxic to nerve cells and may damage or destroy them either in the brain or the peripheral nervous system.

Does Drug Abuse Cause Mental Disorders, or Vice Versa?

Drug abuse and mental disorders often co-exist. In some cases, mental diseases may precede addiction; in other cases, drug abuse may trigger or exacerbate mental disorders, particularly in individuals with specific vulnerabilities.

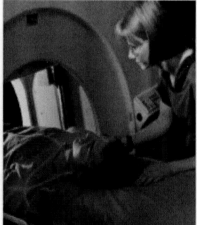

THE IMPACT OF ADDICTION CAN BE FAR REACHING

- Cardiovascular disease
- Stroke
- Cancer
- HIV/AIDS
- Hepatitis B and C
- Lung disease
- Mental disorders

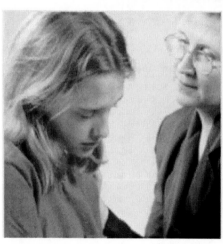

How Can Addiction Harm other People?

Beyond the harmful consequences for the addicted individual, drug abuse can cause serious health problems for others. Three of the more devastating and troubling consequences of addiction are:

Negative Effects of Prenatal Drug Exposure on Infants and Children

It is likely that some drug-exposed children will need educational support in the classroom to help them overcome what may be subtle deficits in developmental areas such as behavior, attention, and cognition. Ongoing work is investigating whether the effects of prenatal exposure on brain and behavior extend into adolescence to cause developmental problems during that time period.

Negative Effects of Second-Hand Smoke

Second-hand tobacco smoke, also referred to as environmental tobacco smoke (ETS), is a significant source of exposure to a large number of substances known to be hazardous to human health, particularly to children. According to the Surgeon General's 2006 Report, The Health Consequences of Involuntary Exposure to Tobacco Smoke, involuntary smoking increases the risk of heart disease and lung cancer in never-smokers by 25–30 percent and 20–30 percent, respectively.

Increased Spread of Infectious Diseases

Injection of drugs such as heroin, cocaine, and methamphetamine accounts for more than a third of new AIDS cases. Injection drug use is also a major factor in the spread of hepatitis C, a serious, potentially fatal liver disease. Injection drug use is not the only way that drug abuse contributes to the spread of infectious diseases. All drugs of abuse cause some form of intoxication, which interferes with judgment and increases the likelihood of risky sexual behaviors. This, in turn, contributes to the spread of HIV/AIDS, hepatitis B and C, and other sexually transmitted diseases.

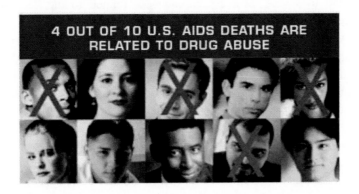

What are Some Effects of Specific Abused Substances

- Nicotine is an addictive stimulant found in cigarettes and other forms of tobacco. Tobacco smoke increases a user's risk of cancer, emphysema, bronchial disorders, and cardiovascular disease. The mortality rate associated with tobacco addiction is staggering. Tobacco use killed approximately 100 million people during the 20th century and, if current smoking trends continue, the cumulative death toll for this century has been projected to reach 1 billion.

- Alcohol consumption can damage the brain and most body organs. Areas of the brain that are especially vulnerable to alcohol-related damage are the cerebral cortex (largely responsible for our higher brain functions, including problemsolving and decisionmaking), the hippocampus (important for memory and learning), and the cerebellum (important for movement coordination).

- Marijuana is the most commonly abused illicit substance. This drug impairs short-term memory and learning, the ability to focus attention, and coordination. It also increases heart rate, can harm the lungs, and can increase the risk of psychosis in those with an underlying vulnerability.

- Inhalants are volatile substances found in many household products, such as oven cleaners, gasoline, spray paints, and other aerosols, that induce mind-altering effects. Inhalants are extremely toxic and can damage the heart, kidneys, lungs, and brain. Even a healthy person can suffer heart failure and death within minutes of a single session of prolonged sniffing of an inhalant.

- Cocaine is a short-acting stimulant, which can lead abusers to "binge" (to take the drug many times in a single session). Cocaine abuse can lead to severe medical consequences related to the heart and the respiratory, nervous, and digestive systems.

- Amphetamines, including methamphetamine, are powerful stimulants that can produce feelings of euphoria and alertness. Methamphetamine's effects are particularly long-lasting and harmful to the brain. Amphetamines can cause high body temperature and can lead to serious heart problems and seizures.

- Ecstasy (MDMA) produces both stimulant and mind-altering effects. It can increase body temperature, heart rate, blood pressure, and heart wall stress. Ecstasy may also be toxic to nerve cells.

- LSD is one of the most potent hallucinogenic, or perception-altering, drugs. Its effects are unpredictable, and abusers may see vivid colors and images, hear sounds, and feel sensations that seem real but do not exist. Abusers also may have traumatic experiences and emotions that can last for many hours. Some short-term effects can include increased body temperature, heart rate, and blood pressure; sweating; loss of appetite; sleeplessness; dry mouth; and tremors.

- Heroin is a powerful opiate drug that produces euphoria and feelings of relaxation. It slows respiration and its use is linked to an increased risk of serious infectious diseases, especially when taken intravenously. Other opioid drugs include morphine, OxyContin, and Vicodin, which have legitimate medical uses; however, their nonmedical use or abuse can result in the same harmful consequences as abusing heroin.

- Prescription medications are increasingly being abused or used for nonmedical purposes. This practice cannot only be addictive, but in some cases also lethal. Commonly abused classes of prescription drugs include painkillers, sedatives, and stimulants. Among the most disturbing aspects of this emerging trend is its prevalence among teenagers and young adults, and the common misperception that because these medications are prescribed by physicians, they are safe even when used illicitly.

- Steroids, which can also be prescribed for certain medical conditions, are abused to increase muscle mass and to improve athletic performance or physical appearance. Serious consequences of abuse can include severe acne, heart disease, liver problems, stroke, infectious diseases, depression, and suicide.

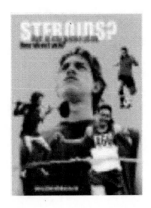

- Drug combinations. A particularly dangerous and not uncommon practice is the combining of two or more drugs. The practice ranges from the co-administration of legal drugs, like alcohol and nicotine, to the dangerous random mixing of prescription drugs, to the deadly combination of heroin or cocaine with fentanyl (an opioid pain medication). Whatever the context, it is critical to realize that because of drug–drug interactions, such practices often pose significantly higher risks than the already harmful individual drugs.

For more information on the nature and extent of common drugs of abuse and their health consequences, go to NIDA's Web site (www.drugabuse.gov) to order free copies of the popular Research Reports (www.drugabuse. gov/ResearchReports/ResearchIndex.html), InfoFacts, and other publications.

V. TREATMENT AND RECOVERY

Can Addiction Be Treated Successfully?

Yes, addiction is a treatable disease. Discoveries in the science of addiction have led to advances in drug abuse treatment that help people stop abusing drugs and resume their productive lives. *Can addiction be cured?*

Addiction need not be a life sentence. Like other chronic diseases, addiction can be managed successfully. Treatment enables people to counteract addiction's powerful disruptive effects on brain and behavior and regain control of their lives.

Does Relapse to Drug Abuse Mean Treatment Has Failed?

No. The chronic nature of the disease means that relapsing to drug abuse is not only possible, but likely. Relapse rates (i.e., how often symptoms recur) for drug addiction are similar to those for other well-characterized chronic medical illnesses such as diabetes, hypertension, and asthma, which also have both physiological and behavioral components. Treatment of chronic diseases involves changing deeply imbedded behaviors, and relapse does not mean treatment failure.

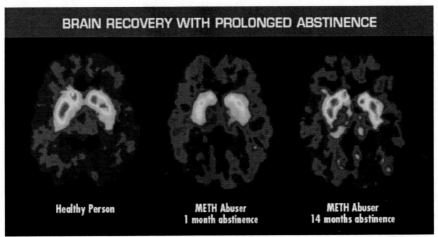

BRAIN RECOVERY WITH PROLONGED ABSTINENCE

Healthy Person   METH Abuser   METH Abuser
                        1 month abstinence   14 months abstinence

Source: J Neurosci 21:9414–9418, 2001.

These images of the dopamine transporter show the brain's remarkable potential to recover, at least partially, after a long abstinence from drugs—in this case, methamphetamine.

For the addicted patient, lapses back to drug abuse indicate that treatment needs to be reinstated or adjusted, or that alternate treatment is needed.

What Are the Principles of Effective Addiction Treatment?

Research shows that combining treatment medications, where available, with behavioral therapy is the best way to ensure success for most patients. Treatment approaches must be tailored to address each patient's drug abuse patterns and drug-related medical, psychiatric, and social problems.

How Can Medications Help Treat Drug Addiction?

Different types of medications may be useful at different stages of treatment to help a patient stop abusing drugs, stay in treatment, and avoid relapse.

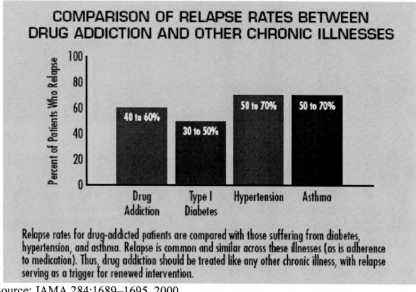

COMPARISON OF RELAPSE RATES BETWEEN DRUG ADDICTION AND OTHER CHRONIC ILLNESSES

Relapse rates for drug-addicted patients are compared with those suffering from diabetes, hypertension, and asthma. Relapse is common and similar across these illnesses (as is adherence to medication). Thus, drug addiction should be treated like any other chronic illness, with relapse serving as a trigger for renewed intervention.

Source: JAMA 284:1689–1695, 2000.

- Treating Withdrawal. When patients first stop abusing drugs, they can experience a variety of physical and emotional symptoms, including depression, anxiety, and other mood disorders; restlessness; and sleeplessness. Certain treatment medications are designed to reduce these symptoms, which makes it easier to stop the abuse.
- Staying in Treatment. Some treatment medications are used to help the brain adapt gradually to the absence of the abused drug. These medications act slowly to stave off drug cravings, and have a calming effect on body systems. They can help patients focus on counseling and other psychotherapies related to their drug treatment.
- Preventing Relapse. Science has taught us that stress, cues linked to the drug experience (e.g., people, places, things, moods), and exposure to drugs are the most common triggers for relapse. Medications are being developed to interfere with these triggers to help patients sustain recovery.

How Do Behavioral Therapies Treat Drug Addiction?

Behavioral treatments help engage people in drug abuse treatment, modifying their attitudes and behaviors related to drug abuse and increasing their life skills to handle stressful circumstances and environmental cues that may trigger intense craving for drugs and prompt another cycle of compulsive abuse. Moreover, behavioral therapies can enhance the effectiveness of medications and help people remain in treatment longer.

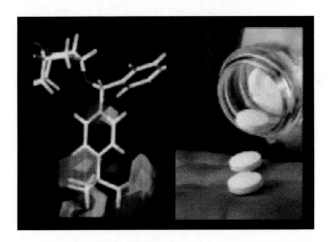

Discoveries in science lead to advances in drug abuse treatment.

MEDICATIONS USED TO TREAT DRUG ADDICTION

- **Tobacco Addiction**
  - Nicotine replacement therapies (e.g., patch, inhaler, gum)
  - Bupropion
  - Varenicline

- **Opioid Addiction**
  - Methadone
  - Buprenorphine
  - Naltrexone

- **Alcohol and Drug Addiction**
  - Naltrexone
  - Disulfiram
  - Acamprosate

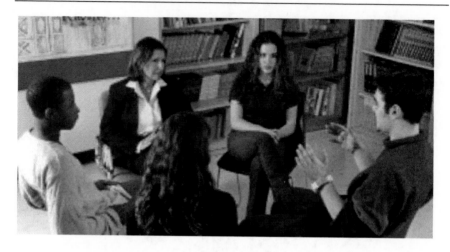

- Cognitive Behavioral Therapy. Seeks to help patients recognize, avoid, and cope with the situations in which they are most likely to abuse drugs.
- Motivational Incentives. Uses positive reinforcement such as providing rewards or privileges for remaining drug free, for attending and participating in counseling sessions, or for taking treatment medications as prescribed.
- Motivational Interviewing. Employs strategies to evoke rapid and internally motivated behavior change to stop drug use and facilitate treatment entry.
- Group Therapy. Helps patients face their drug abuse realistically, come to terms with its harmful consequences, and boost their motivation to stay drug free. Patients learn effective ways to solve their emotional and interpersonal problems without resorting to drugs.

How Do the Best Treatment Programs Help Patients Recover from the Pervasive Effects of Addiction?

Getting an addicted person to stop abusing drugs is just one part of a long and complex recovery process. When people enter treatment, addiction has often taken over their lives. The compulsion to get drugs, take drugs, and experience the effects of drugs has dominated their every waking moment, and drug abuse has taken the place of all the things they used to enjoy doing. It has disrupted how they function in their family lives, at work, and in the community, and has made them more likely to suffer from other serious illnesses. Because addiction can affect so many aspects of a person's life, treatment must address the needs of the whole person to be successful. This is why the best programs incorporate a variety of rehabilitative services into their comprehensive treatment regimens. Treatment counselors select from a menu of services for meeting the individual medical, psychological, social, vocational, and legal needs of their patients to foster their recovery from addiction.

For more information on drug treatment, see Principles of Drug Addiction Treatment: A Research-Based Guide (www.drugabuse.gov/PODAT/PODA TIndex.html).

VI. ADVANCING ADDICTION SCIENCE AND PRACTICAL SOLUTIONS

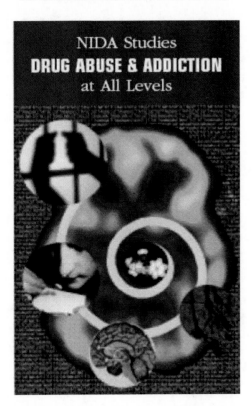

Leading the Search for Scientific Solutions

To address all aspects of drug abuse and its harmful consequences, NIDA's research program ranges from basic studies of the addicted brain and behavior to health services research. NIDA's research program develops prevention and treatment approaches and ensures they work in real-world settings. In this context, NIDA is strongly committed to developing a research portfolio that addresses the special vulnerabilities and health disparities that exist among ethnic minorities or that derive from gender differences.

Bringing Science to Real-World Settings

National Drug Abuse Treatment Clinical Trials Network (CTN)
The CTN "road tests" research-based drug abuse treatments in community treatment programs around the country.

Criminal Justice Drug Abuse Treatment Studies (CJ-DATS)
Led by NIDA, CJ-DATS is a network of research centers, in partnership with criminal justice professionals, drug abuse treatment providers, and Federal agencies responsible for developing integrated treatment approaches for criminal justice offenders and testing them at multiple sites throughout the Nation.

Sharing Free Information with the Public

NIDA further increases the impact of its research on the problems of addiction by sharing free information about its findings with professional audiences and the general public. Special initiatives target students and teachers, designated populations, and ethnic groups.

In: Drug Addiction: Science and Treatment   ISBN: 978-1-61470-004-3
Editors: N. Jacobs and L. C. Dubois   © 2012 Nova Science Publishers, Inc.

Chapter 2

PRINCIPLES OF DRUG ADDICTION TREATMENT: A RESEARCH-BASED GUIDE[*]

National Institute on Drug Abuse

PREFACE

Drug addiction is a complex illness. It is characterized by intense and, at times, uncontrollable drug craving, along with compulsive drug seeking and use that persist even in the face of devastating consequences.

Many people do not realize that addiction is a brain disease. While the path to drug addiction begins with the act of taking drugs, over time a person's ability to choose not to do so becomes compromised, and seeking and consuming the drug becomes compulsive. This behavior results largely from the effects of prolonged drug exposure on brain functioning. Addiction affects multiple brain circuits, including those involved in reward and motivation, learning and memory, and inhibitory control over behavior. Some individuals are more vulnerable than others to becoming addicted, depending on genetic makeup, age of exposure to drugs, other environmental influences, and the interplay of all these factors.

Addiction is often more than just compulsive drug taking—it can also produce far-reaching consequences. For example, drug abuse and addiction

---

[*] This is an edited, reformatted and augmented version of a National Institute on Drug Abuse publication, second edition, dated October 1999; Reprinted July 2000, February 2008; Revised April 2009.

increase a person's risk for a variety of other mental and physical illnesses related to a drug-abusing lifestyle or the toxic effects of the drugs themselves. Additionally, a wide range of dysfunctional behaviors can result from drug abuse and interfere with normal functioning in the family, the workplace, and the broader community.

Because drug abuse and addiction have so many dimensions and disrupt so many aspects of an individual's life, treatment is not simple. Effective treatment programs typically incorporate many components, each directed to a particular aspect of the illness and its consequences. Addiction treatment must help the individual stop using drugs, maintain a drug-free lifestyle, and achieve productive functioning in the family, at work, and in society. Because addiction is a disease, people cannot simply stop using drugs for a few days and be cured. Most patients require long-term or repeated episodes of care to achieve the ultimate goal of sustained abstinence and recovery of their lives.

Indeed, scientific research and clinical practice demonstrate the value of continuing care in treating addiction, with a variety of approaches having been tested and integrated in residential and community settings. As we look toward the future, we will harness new research results on the influence of genetics and environment on gene function and expression (i.e., epigenetics), which are heralding the development of personalized treatment interventions. These findings will be integrated with current evidence supporting the most effective drug abuse and addiction treatments and their implementation, which are reflected in this guide.

This update of the National Institute on Drug Abuse's *Principles of Drug Addiction Treatment* is intended to address addiction to a wide variety of drugs, including nicotine, alcohol, and illicit and prescription drugs. It is designed to serve as a resource for health care providers, family members, and other stakeholders trying to address the myriad problems faced by patients in need of treatment for drug abuse or addiction.

Nora D. Volkow, M.D.
Director
National Institute on Drug Abuse

PRINCIPLES OF EFFECTIVE TREATMENT

1) *Addiction is a complex but treatable disease that affects brain function and behavior.* Drugs of abuse alter the brain's structure and function, resulting in changes that persist long after drug use has ceased. This may explain why drug abusers are at risk for relapse even after long periods of abstinence and despite the potentially devastating consequences.

2) *No single treatment is appropriate for everyone.* Matching treatment settings, interventions, and services to an individual's particular problems and needs is critical to his or her ultimate success in returning to productive functioning in the family, workplace, and society.

3) *Treatment needs to be readily available.* Because drug-addicted individuals may be uncertain about entering treatment, taking advantage of available services the moment people are ready for treatment is critical. Potential patients can be lost if treatment is not immediately available or readily accessible. As with other chronic diseases, the earlier treatment is offered in the disease process, the greater the likelihood of positive outcomes.

4) *Effective treatment attends to multiple needs of the individual, not just his or her drug abuse.* To be effective, treatment must address the individual's drug abuse and any associated medical, psychological, social, vocational, and legal problems. It is also important that treatment be appropriate to the individual's age, gender, ethnicity, and culture.

5) *Remaining in treatment for an adequate period of time is critical.* The appropriate duration for an individual depends on the type and degree of his or her problems and needs. Research indicates that most addicted individuals need at least 3 months in treatment to significantly reduce or stop their drug use and that the best outcomes occur with longer durations of treatment. Recovery from drug addiction is a long-term process and frequently requires multiple episodes of treatment. As with other chronic illnesses, relapses to drug abuse can occur and should signal a need for treatment to be reinstated or adjusted. Because individuals often leave treatment prematurely, programs should include strategies to engage and keep patients in treatment.

6) *Counseling—individual and/or group— and other behavioral therapies are the most commonly used forms of drug abuse treatment.* Behavioral therapies vary in their focus and may involve addressing a patient's motivation to change, providing incentives for abstinence, building skills to resist drug use, replacing drug-using activities with constructive and rewarding activities, improving problem solving skills, and facilitating better interpersonal relationships. Also, participation in group therapy and other peer support programs during and following treatment can help maintain abstinence.

7) *Medications are an important element of treatment for many patients, especially when combined with counseling and other behavioral therapies.* For example, methadone and buprenorphine are effective in helping individuals addicted to heroin or other opioids stabilize their lives and reduce their illicit drug use. Naltrexone is also an effective medication for some opioid-addicted individuals and some patients with alcohol dependence. Other medications for alcohol dependence include acamprosate, disulfiram, and topiramate. For persons addicted to nicotine, a nicotine replacement product (such as patches, gum, or lozenges) or an oral medication (such as bupropion or varenicline) can be an effective component of treatment when part of a comprehensive behavioral treatment program.

8) *An individual's treatment and services plan must be assessed continually and modified as necessary to ensure that it meets his or her changing needs.* A patient may require varying combinations of services and treatment components during the course of treatment and recovery. In addition to counseling or psychotherapy, a patient may require medication, medical services, family therapy, parenting instruction, vocational rehabilitation, and/or social and legal services. For many patients, a continuing care approach provides the best results, with the treatment intensity varying according to a person's changing needs.

9) *Many drug-addicted individuals also have other mental disorders.* Because drug abuse and addiction—both of which are mental disorders—often co-occur with other mental illnesses, patients presenting with one condition should be assessed for the other(s). And when these problems co-occur, treatment should address both (or all), including the use of medications as appropriate.

10) *Medically assisted detoxification is only the first stage of addiction treatment and by itself does little to change long-term drug abuse.*

Although medically assisted detoxification can safely manage the acute physical symptoms of withdrawal and, for some, can pave the way for effective long-term addiction treatment, detoxification alone is rarely sufficient to help addicted individuals achieve long-term abstinence. Thus, patients should be encouraged to continue drug treatment following detoxification. Motivational enhancement and incentive strategies, begun at initial patient intake, can improve treatment engagement.

11) *Treatment does not need to be voluntary to be effective.* Sanctions or enticements from family, employment settings, and/or the criminal justice system can significantly increase treatment entry, retention rates, and the ultimate success of drug treatment interventions.

12) *Drug use during treatment must be monitored continuously, as lapses during treatment do occur.* Knowing their drug use is being monitored can be a powerful incentive for patients and can help them withstand urges to use drugs. Monitoring also provides an early indication of a return to drug use, signaling a possible need to adjust an individual's treatment plan to better meet his or her needs.

13) *Treatment programs should assess patients for the presence of HIV/ AIDS, hepatitis B and C, tuberculosis, and other infectious diseases as well as provide targeted risk-reduction counseling to help patients modify or change behaviors that place them at risk of contracting or spreading infectious diseases.* Typically, drug abuse treatment addresses some of the drug-related behaviors that put people at risk of infectious diseases. Targeted counseling specifically focused on reducing infectious disease risk can help patients further reduce or avoid substance-related and other high-risk behaviors. Counseling can also help those who are already infected to manage their illness. Moreover, engaging in substance abuse treatment can facilitate adherence to other medical treatments. Patients may be reluctant to accept screening for HIV (and other infectious diseases); therefore, it is incumbent upon treatment providers to encourage and support HIV screening and inform patients that highly active antiretroviral therapy (HAART) has proven effective in combating HIV, including among drug-abusing populations.

FREQUENTLY ASKED QUESTIONS

1. Why Do Drug-Addicted Persons Keep Using Drugs?

Nearly all addicted individuals believe at the outset that they can stop using drugs on their own, and most try to stop without treatment. Although some people are successful, many attempts result in failure to achieve long-term abstinence. Research has shown that long-term drug abuse results in changes in the brain that persist long after a person stops using drugs. These drug-induced changes in brain function can have many behavioral consequences, including an inability to exert control over the impulse to use drugs despite adverse consequences—the defining characteristic of addiction.

Understanding that addiction has such a fundamental biological component may help explain the difficulty of achieving and maintaining abstinence without treatment. Psychological stress from work, family problems, psychiatric illness, pain associated with medical problems, social cues (such as meeting individuals from one's drug-using past), or environmental cues (such as encountering streets, objects, or even smells associated with drug abuse) can trigger intense cravings without the individual even being consciously aware of the triggering event. Any one of these factors can hinder attainment of sustained abstinence and make relapse more likely. Nevertheless, research indicates that active participation in treatment is an essential component for good outcomes and can benefit even the most severely addicted individuals.

> *Long-term drug use results in significant changes in brain function that can persist long after the individual stops using drugs.*

 ## 2. What Is Drug Addiction Treatment?

Drug treatment is intended to help addicted individuals stop compulsive drug seeking and use. Treatment can occur in a variety of settings, in many different forms, and for different lengths of time. Because drug addiction is typically a chronic disorder characterized by occasional relapses, a short-term, one-time treatment is usually not sufficient. For many, treatment is a long-term process that involves multiple interventions and regular monitoring.

Components of Comprehensive Drug Abuse Treatment

CHILD CARE SERVICES

FAMILY SERVICES

VOCATIONAL SERVICES

HOUSING / TRANSPORTATION SERVICES

MENTAL HEALTH SERVICES

INTAKE PROCESSING/ ASSESSMENT

BEHAVIORAL THERAPY AND COUNSELING | TREATMENT PLAN | SUBSTANCE USE MONITORING

FINANCIAL SERVICES

CLINICAL AND CASE MANAGEMENT | PHARMACOTHERAPY | SELF-HELP/PEER SUPPORT GROUPS

MEDICAL SERVICES

CONTINUING CARE

LEGAL SERVICES

EDUCATIONAL SERVICES

HIV/AIDS SERVICES

The best treatment programs provide a combination of therapies and other services to meet the needs of the individual patient.

There are a variety of evidence-based approaches to treating addiction. Drug treatment can include behavioral therapy (such as individual or group counseling, cognitive therapy, or contingency management), medications, or their combination. The specific type of treatment or combination of treatments will vary depending on the patient's individual needs and, often, on the types of drugs they use. The severity of addiction and previous efforts to stop using drugs can also influence a treatment approach. Finally, people who are addicted to drugs often suffer from other health (including other mental health), occupational, legal, familial, and social problems that should be addressed concurrently.

The best programs provide a combination of therapies and other services to meet an individual patient's needs. Specific needs may relate to age, race, culture, sexual orientation, gender, pregnancy, other drug use, comorbid conditions (e.g., depression, HIV), parenting, housing, and employment, as well as physical and sexual abuse history.

Drug addiction treatment can include medications, behavioral therapies, or their combination.

Treatment medications, such as methadone, buprenorphine, and naltrexone, are available for individuals addicted to opioids, while nicotine preparations (patches, gum, lozenges, and nasal spray) and the medications varenicline and bupropion are available for individuals addicted to tobacco. Disulfiram, acamprosate, naltrexone, and topiramate are medications used for treating alcohol dependence, which commonly co-occurs with other drug addictions. In fact, most people with severe addiction are polydrug users and require treatment for all substances abused. Even combined alcohol and tobacco use has proven amenable to concurrent treatment for both substances.

Psychoactive medications, such as antidepressants, antianxiety agents, mood stabilizers, and antipsychotic medications, may be critical for treatment success when patients have co-occurring mental disorders, such as depression, anxiety disorders (including post-traumatic stress disorder), bipolar disorder, or schizophrenia.

Behavioral therapies can help motivate people to participate in drug treatment; offer strategies for coping with drug cravings; teach ways to avoid drugs and prevent relapse; and help individuals deal with relapse if it occurs. Behavioral therapies can also help people improve communication, relationship, and parenting skills, as well as family dynamics.

Many treatment programs employ both individual and group therapies. Group therapy can provide social reinforcement and help enforce behavioral contingencies that promote abstinence and a non-drugusing lifestyle. Some of the more established behavioral treatments, such as contingency management and cognitive-behavioral therapy, are also being adapted for group settings to improve efficiency and cost-effectiveness. However, particularly in adolescents, there can also be a danger of iatrogenic, or inadvertent, effects of group treatment; thus, trained counselors should be aware and monitor for such effects.

Because they work on different aspects of addiction, combinations of behavioral therapies and medications (when available) generally appear to be more effective than either approach used alone.

Treatment for drug abuse and addiction is delivered in many different settings using a variety of behavioral and pharmacological approaches.

*Comparison of Relapse Rates between Drug Addiction
and other Chronic Illnesses*

Percentage of Patients Who Relapse

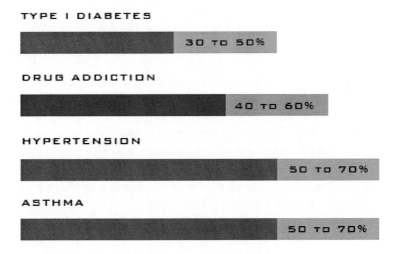

TYPE I DIABETES
30 TO 50%

DRUG ADDICTION
40 TO 60%

HYPERTENSION
50 TO 70%

ASTHMA
50 TO 70%

3. How Effective Is Drug Addiction Treatment?

In addition to stopping drug abuse, the goal of treatment is to return people to productive functioning in the family, workplace, and community. According to research that tracks individuals in treatment over extended periods, most people who get into and remain in treatment stop using drugs, decrease their criminal activity, and improve their occupational, social, and psychological functioning. For example, methadone treatment has been shown to increase participation in behavioral therapy and decrease both drug use and criminal behavior. However, individual treatment outcomes depend on the extent and nature of the patient's problems, the appropriateness of treatment and related services used to address those problems, and the quality of interaction between the patient and his or her treatment providers.

> *Relapse rates for addiction resemble those of other chronic diseases such as diabetes, hypertension, and asthma.*

Like other chronic diseases, addiction can be managed successfully. Treatment enables people to counteract addiction's powerful disruptive effects on the brain and behavior and to regain control of their lives. The chronic nature of the disease means that relapsing to drug abuse is not only possible but also likely, with relapse rates similar to those for other well-characterized chronic medical illnesses—such as diabetes, hypertension, and asthma (see figure, "Comparison of Relapse Rates Between Drug Addiction and Other Chronic Illnesses")—that also have both physiological and behavioral components.

Unfortunately, when relapse occurs many deem treatment a failure. This is not the case: successful treatment for addiction typically requires continual evaluation and modification as appropriate, similar to the approach taken for other chronic diseases. For example, when a patient is receiving active treatment for hypertension and symptoms decrease, treatment is deemed successful, even though symptoms may recur when treatment is discontinued. For the addicted patient, lapses to drug abuse do not indicate failure—rather, they signify that treatment needs to be reinstated or adjusted, or that alternate treatment is needed (see figure, "How Do We Evaluate if a Treatment is Effective?").

4. Is Drug Addiction Treatment Worth its Cost?

Substance abuse costs our Nation over one half-trillion dollars annually, and treatment can help reduce these costs. Drug addiction treatment has been shown to reduce associated health and social costs by far more than the cost of the treatment itself. Treatment is also much less expensive than its alternatives, such as incarcerating addicted persons. For example, the average cost for 1 full year of methadone maintenance treatment is approximately $4,700 per patient, whereas 1 full year of imprisonment costs approximately $24,000 per person.

According to several conservative estimates, every $1 invested in addiction treatment programs yields a return of between $4 and $7 in reduced drug-related crime, criminal justice costs, and theft. When savings related to health care are included, total savings can exceed costs by a ratio of 12 to 1.

> *Drug addiction treatment reduces drug use and its associated health and social costs.*

How Do We Evaluate if a Treatment is Effective?

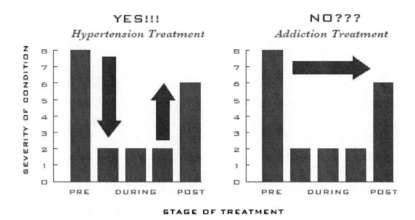

Major savings to the individual and to society also stem from fewer interpersonal conflicts; greater workplace productivity; and fewer drug-related accidents, including overdoses and deaths.

5. How Long Does Drug Addiction Treatment Usually Last?

Individuals progress through drug addiction treatment at various rates, so there is no predetermined length of treatment. However, research has shown unequivocally that good outcomes are contingent on adequate treatment length. Generally, for residential or outpatient treatment, participation for less than 90 days is of limited effectiveness, and treatment lasting significantly longer is recommended for maintaining positive outcomes. For methadone maintenance, 12 months is considered the minimum, and some opioid addicted individuals continue to benefit from methadone maintenance for many years.

Treatment dropout is one of the major problems encountered by treatment programs; therefore, motivational techniques that can keep patients engaged will also improve outcomes. By viewing addiction as a chronic disease and offering continuing care and monitoring, programs can succeed, but this will often require multiple episodes of treatment and readily readmitting patients that have relapsed.

> *Good outcomes are contingent on adequate treatment length.*

6. What Helps People Stay in Treatment?

Because successful outcomes often depend on a person's staying in treatment long enough to reap its full benefits, strategies for keeping people in treatment are critical. Whether a patient stays in treatment depends on factors associated with both the individual and the program. Individual factors related to engagement and retention typically include motivation to change drug-using behavior; degree of support from family and friends; and, frequently, pressure from the criminal justice system, child protection services, employers, or the family. Within a treatment program, successful clinicians can establish a positive, therapeutic relationship with their patients. The clinician should ensure that a treatment plan is developed cooperatively with the person seeking treatment, that the plan is followed, and that treatment expectations are clearly understood. Medical, psychiatric, and social services should also be available.

Because some problems (such as serious medical or mental illness or criminal involvement) increase the likelihood of patients dropping out of treatment, intensive interventions may be required to retain them. After a course of intensive treatment, the provider should ensure a transition to less intensive continuing care to support and monitor individuals in their ongoing recovery.

> *Whether a patient stays in treatment depends on factors associated with both the individual and the program.*

7. How Do We Get More Substance-Abusing People into Treatment?

It has been known for many years that the "treatment gap" is massive—that is, among those who need treatment for a substance use disorder, few receive it. In 2007, 23.2 million persons aged 12 or older needed treatment for an illicit drug or alcohol use problem, but only 3.9 million received treatment at a specialty substance abuse facility.

Reducing this gap requires a multipronged approach. Strategies include increasing access to effective treatment, achieving insurance parity (now in its earliest phase of implementation), reducing stigma, and raising awareness among both patients and health care professionals of the value of addiction treatment. To assist physicians in identifying treatment need in their patients and making appropriate referrals, NIDA is encouraging widespread use of screening, brief intervention, and referral to treatment (SBIRT) tools for use in primary care settings. SBIRT— which has proven effective against tobacco and alcohol use— has the potential not only to catch people before serious drug problems develop but also to connect them with appropriate treatment providers.

8. How Can Families and Friends Make a Difference in the Life of Someone Needing Treatment?

Family and friends can play critical roles in motivating individuals with drug problems to enter and stay in treatment. Family therapy can also be important, especially for adolescents. Involvement of a family member or significant other in an individual's treatment program can strengthen and extend treatment benefits.

9. Where Can Family Members Go for Information on Treatment Options?

Trying to locate appropriate treatment for a loved one, especially finding a program tailored to an individual's particular needs, can be a difficult process. However, there are some resources currently available to help with this process, including—

- The Substance Abuse and Mental Health Services Administration (SAMHSA) maintains a Web site (www.findtreatment.samhsa.gov) that shows the location of residential, outpatient, and hospital inpatient treatment programs for drug addiction and alcoholism throughout the country. This information is also accessible by calling 1-800-662-HELP.
- The National Suicide Prevention Lifeline (1-800-273-TALK) offers more than just suicide prevention—it can also help with a host of issues, including drug and alcohol abuse, and can connect individuals with a nearby professional.
- The National Alliance on Mental Illness (www.nami.org) and Mental Health America (www.mentalhealthamerica.net) are alliances of nonprofit, self-help support organizations for patients and families

dealing with a variety of mental disorders. Both have State and local affiliates throughout the country and may be especially helpful for patients with comorbid conditions.

- The American Academy of Addiction Psychiatry and the American Academy of Child and Adolescent Psychiatry each have physician locator tools posted on their Web sites at www.aaap.org and www.aacap.org, respectively.

- For information about participating in a clinical trial testing promising substance abuse interventions, contact NIDA's National Drug Abuse Treatment Clinical Trials Network at www.drugabuse.gov/CTN/Index.htm, or visit NIH's Web site at www.clinicaltrials.gov.

10. How Can the Workplace Play a Role in Substance Abuse Treatment?

Many workplaces sponsor Employee Assistance Programs (EAPs) that offer short-term counseling and/or assistance in linking employees with drug or alcohol problems to local treatment resources, including peer support/recovery groups. In addition, therapeutic work environments that provide employment for drug-abusing individuals who can demonstrate abstinence have been shown not only to promote a continued drug-free lifestyle but also to improve job skills, punctuality, and other behaviors necessary for active employment throughout life. Urine testing facilities, trained personnel, and workplace monitors are needed to implement this type of treatment.

11. What Role Can the Criminal Justice System Play in Addressing Drug Addiction?

Research has demonstrated that treatment for drug-addicted offenders during and after incarceration can have a significant effect on future drug use, criminal behavior, and social functioning. The case for integrating drug addiction treatment approaches with the criminal justice system is compelling. Combining prison- and community-based treatment for addicted offenders reduces the risk of both recidivism to drug-related criminal behavior and relapse to drug use, which, in turn, nets huge savings in societal costs. One study found that prisoners who participated in a therapeutic treatment program in the Delaware State prison system and continued to receive treatment in a work-release program after prison were 70 percent less likely than nonparticipants to return to drug use and incur re-arrest.

The majority of offenders involved with the criminal justice system are not in prison but are under community supervision. For those with known drug problems, drug addiction treatment may be recommended or mandated as a condition of probation. Research has demonstrated that individuals who enter treatment under legal pressure have outcomes as favorable as those who enter treatment voluntarily.

The criminal justice system refers drug offenders into treatment through a variety of mechanisms, such as diverting nonviolent offenders to treatment; stipulating treatment as a condition of incarceration, probation, or pretrial release; and convening specialized courts, or drug courts, that handle drug offense cases. These courts mandate and arrange for treatment as an alternative to incarceration, actively monitor progress in treatment, and arrange for other services for drug-involved offenders.

The most effective models integrate criminal justice and drug treatment systems and services. Treatment and criminal justice personnel work together on treatment planning—including implementation of screening, placement, testing, monitoring, and supervision—as well as on the systematic use of sanctions and rewards.

Treatment for incarcerated drug abusers should include continuing care, monitoring, and supervision after incarceration and during parole. (For more information, please see NIDA's Principles of Drug Abuse Treatment for Criminal Justice Populations: A Research-Based Guide [revised 2007].)

Individuals who enter treatment under legal pressure have outcomes as favorable as those who enter treatment voluntarily.

12. What Are the Unique Needs of Women with Substance Use Disorders?

Gender-related drug abuse treatment should attend not only to biological differences but also to social and environmental factors, all of which can influence the motivations for drug use, the reasons for seeking treatment, the types of environments where treatment is obtained, the treatments that are most effective, and the consequences of not receiving treatment. Many life circumstances predominate in women as a group, which may require a specialized treatment approach. For example, research has shown that physical and sexual trauma followed by post-traumatic stress disorder (PTSD) is more common in drug-abusing women than in men seeking treatment. Other factors unique to women that can influence the treatment process include issues around pregnancy and child care, financial independence, and how they come into treatment (as women are more likely to seek the assistance of a general or mental health practitioner).

13. What Are the Unique Needs of Adolescents with Substance Use Disorders?

Adolescent drug abusers have unique needs stemming from their immature neurocognitive and psychosocial stage of development. Research has demonstrated that the brain undergoes a prolonged process of development and refinement, from birth to early adulthood, during which a developmental shift occurs where actions go from more impulsive to more reasoned and reflective.

In fact, the brain areas most closely associated with aspects of behavior such as decisionmaking, judgment, planning, and self-control undergo a period of rapid development during adolescence.

Adolescent drug abuse is also often associated with other co-occurring mental health problems. These include attention-deficit hyperactivity disorder (ADHD), oppositional defiant disorder, and conduct problems, as well as depressive and anxiety disorders. This developmental period has also been associated with physical and/or sexual abuse and academic difficulties.

Adolescents are also especially sensitive to social cues, with peer groups and families being highly influential during this time. Therefore, treatments that facilitate positive parental involvement, integrate other systems in which the adolescent participates (such as school and athletics), and recognize the importance of prosocial peer relationships are among the most effective. Access to comprehensive assessment, treatment, case management, and family-support services that are developmentally, culturally, and gender-appropriate is also integral when addressing adolescent addiction.

Medications for substance abuse among adolescents may also be helpful. Currently, the only Food and Drug Administration (FDA)-approved addiction medication for adolescents is the transdermal nicotine patch. Research is under way to determine the safety and efficacy of medications for nicotine-, alcohol-, and opioid-dependent adolescents and for adolescents with co-occurring disorders.

14. Are there Specific Drug Addiction Treatments for Older Adults?

With the aging of the baby boomer generation, the composition of the general population will expand dramatically with respect to the number of older adults. Such a change, coupled with a greater history of lifetime drug use (than previous older generations), different cultural norms and general attitudes about drug use, and increases in the availability of psychotherapeutic medications, may lead to growth in the number of older adults with substance use problems. Although no drug treatment programs are yet designed exclusively for older adults, research to date indicates that current addiction treatment programs can be as effective for older adults as they are for younger adults. However, substance abuse problems in older adults often go unrecognized, and therefore untreated.

15. Are there Treatments for People Addicted to Prescription Drugs?

The nonmedical use of prescription drugs increased dramatically in the 1990s and remains at high levels. In 2007, approximately 7 million people aged 12 or older reported nonmedical use of a prescription drug. The most commonly abused medications are painkillers (i.e., opioids: 5.2 million people), stimulants (e.g., methylphenidate and amphetamine: 1.2 million), and central nervous system (CNS) depressants (e.g., benzodiazepines: 2.1 million). Like many illicit substances, these drugs alter the brain's activity and can lead to many adverse consequences, including addiction. For example, opioid pain relievers, such as Vicodin or OxyContin, can present similar health risks as do illicit opioids (e.g., heroin) depending on dose, route of administration, combination with other drugs, and other factors. As a result, the increases in nonmedical use have been accompanied by increased emergency room visits, accidental poisonings, and treatment admissions for addiction. Treatments for prescription drugs tend to be similar to those for illicit drugs that affect the same brain systems. Thus, buprenorphine is used to treat addiction to opioid pain medications, and behavioral therapies are most likely to be effective for stimulant or CNS depressant addiction—for which we do not yet have medications.

16. Is there a Difference between Physical Dependence and Addiction?

Yes. According to the DSM, the clinical criteria for "drug dependence" (or what we refer to as addiction) include compulsive drug use despite harmful consequences; inability to stop using a drug; failure to meet work, social, or family obligations; and, sometimes (depending on the drug), tolerance and withdrawal. The latter reflect physical dependence in which the body adapts to the drug, requiring more of it to achieve a certain effect (tolerance) and eliciting drug-specific physical or mental symptoms if drug use is abruptly ceased (withdrawal). Physical dependence can happen with the chronic use of many drugs—including even appropriate, medically instructed use. Thus, physical dependence in and of itself does not constitute addiction, but often accompanies addiction. This distinction can be difficult to discern, particularly with prescribed pain medications, where the need for increasing dosages can represent tolerance or a worsening underlying problem, as opposed to the beginning of abuse or addiction.

17. Can a Person Become Addicted to Psychotherapeutics that Are Prescribed by a Doctor?

While this scenario occurs infrequently, it is possible. Because some psychotherapeutics have a risk of addiction associated with them (e.g., stimulants to treat ADHD, benzodiazepines to treat anxiety or sleep disorders, and opioids to treat pain), it is important for patients to follow their physician's instructions faithfully and for physicians to monitor their patients carefully. To minimize these risks, a physician (or other prescribing health provider) should be aware of a patient's prior or current substance abuse problems, as well as their family history with regard to addiction. This will help determine risk and need for monitoring.

18. How Do other Mental Disorders Coexisting with Drug Addiction Affect Drug Addiction Treatment?

Drug addiction is a disease of the brain that frequently occurs with other mental disorders. In fact, as many as 6 in 10 people with an illicit substance use disorder also suffer from another mental illness; and rates are similar for users of licit drugs—i.e., tobacco and alcohol. For these individuals, one condition becomes more difficult to treat successfully as an additional condition is intertwined. Thus, patients entering treatment either for a substance use disorder or for another mental disorder should be assessed for the co-occurrence of the other condition. Research indicates that treating both (or multiple) illnesses simultaneously in an integrated fashion is generally the best treatment approach for these patients.

19. Is the Use of Medications Like Methadone and Buprenorphine Simply Replacing One Drug Addiction with Another?

No—as used in maintenance treatment, buprenorphine and methadone are not heroin/opioid substitutes. They are prescribed or administered under monitored, controlled conditions and are safe and effective for treating opioid addiction when used as directed. They are administered orally or sublingually (i.e., under the tongue) in specified doses, and their pharmacological effects differ from those of heroin and other abused opioids.

Heroin, for example, is often injected, snorted, or smoked, causing an almost immediate "rush," or brief period of euphoria, that wears off quickly and ends in a "crash." The individual then experiences an intense craving to use again so as to stop the crash and reinstate the euphoria.

The cycle of euphoria, crash, and craving—sometimes repeated several times a day—is a hallmark of addiction and results in severe behavioral disruption. These characteristics result from heroin's rapid onset and short duration of action in the brain.

In contrast, methadone and buprenorphine have gradual onsets of action and produce stable levels of the drug in the brain; as a result, patients maintained on these medications do not experience a rush, while they also markedly reduce their desire to use opioids. If an individual treated with these medications tries to take an opioid such as heroin, the euphoric effects are usually dampened or suppressed. Patients undergoing maintenance treatment do not experience the physiological or behavioral abnormalities from rapid fluctuations in drug levels associated with heroin use. Maintenance treatments save lives—they help to stabilize individuals, allowing treatment of their medical, psychological, and other problems so they can contribute effectively as members of families and of society.

> *As used in maintenance treatment, methadone and buprenorphine are not heroin/opioid substitutes.*

20. Where Do 12-Step or Self-Help Programs Fit into Drug Addiction Treatment?

Self-help groups can complement and extend the effects of professional treatment. The most prominent self-help groups are those affiliated with Alcoholics Anonymous (AA), Narcotics Anonymous (NA), and Cocaine Anonymous (CA), all of which are based on the 12-step model. Most drug addiction treatment programs encourage patients to participate in self-help group therapy during and after formal treatment. These groups can be particularly helpful during recovery, offering an added layer of community-level social support to help people achieve and maintain abstinence and other healthy lifestyle behaviors over the course of a lifetime.

21. Can Exercise Play a Role in the Treatment Process?

Yes—exercise is increasingly becoming a component of many treatment programs and has shown efficacy, in combination with cognitive-behavioral therapy, for promoting smoking cessation. Exercise may exert beneficial effects by addressing psychosocial and physiological needs that nicotine replacement alone does not; attenuating negative affect; reducing stress; and helping prevent weight gain following cessation. Research is currently under way to determine if and how exercise programs can play a similar role in the treatment of other forms of drug abuse.

22. How Does Drug Addiction Treatment Help Reduce the Spread of HIV/AIDS, Hepatitis C (HCV), and other Infectious Diseases?

Drug-abusing individuals, including injecting and non-injecting drug users, are at increased risk of HIV, HCV, and other infectious diseases. These diseases are transmitted by sharing contaminated drug injection equipment and by engaging in risky sexual behavior sometimes associated with drug use. Effective drug abuse treatment is HIV/HCV prevention because it reduces associated risk behaviors as well as drug abuse. Counseling that targets a range of HIV/HCV risk behaviors provides an added level of disease prevention.

Drug injectors who do not enter treatment are up to six times more likely to become infected with HIV than injectors who enter and remain in treatment because the latter reduce activities that can spread disease, such as sharing injection equipment and engaging in unprotected sexual activity. Participation in treatment also presents opportunities for screening, counseling, and referral to additional services, including early HIV treatment and access to HAART. In fact, HIV counseling and testing are key aspects of superior drug abuse treatment programs and should be offered to all individuals entering treatment.

Greater availability of inexpensive and unobtrusive rapid HIV tests should increase access to these important aspects of HIV prevention and treatment.

> *Drug abuse treatment is HIV and HCV prevention.*

DRUG ADDICTION TREATMENT IN THE UNITED STATES

Drug addiction is a complex disorder that can involve virtually every aspect of an individual's functioning: in the family, at work and school, and in the community. Because of addiction's complexity and pervasive consequences, drug addiction treatment typically must involve many components. Some of those components focus directly on the individual's drug use; others, like employment training, focus on restoring the addicted individual to productive membership in the family and society (see diagram on page 8), enabling him or her to experience the rewards associated with abstinence.

Treatment for drug abuse and addiction is delivered in many different settings using a variety of behavioral and pharmacological approaches. In the United States, more than 13,000 specialized drug treatment facilities provide counseling, behavioral therapy, medication, case management, and other types of services to persons with substance use disorders.

Along with specialized drug treatment facilities, drug abuse and addiction are treated in physicians' offices and mental health clinics by a variety of providers, including counselors, physicians, psychiatrists, psychologists, nurses, and social workers. Treatment is delivered in outpatient, inpatient, and residential settings. Although specific treatment approaches often are associated with particular treatment settings, a variety of therapeutic interventions or services can be included in any given setting.

Because drug abuse and addiction are major public health problems, a large portion of drug treatment is funded by local, State, and Federal governments. Private and employer-subsidized health plans also may provide coverage for treatment of addiction and its medical consequences. Unfortunately, managed care has resulted in shorter average stays, while a historical lack of or insufficient coverage for substance abuse treatment has curtailed the number of operational programs. The recent passage of parity for insurance coverage of mental health and substance abuse problems will hopefully improve this state of affairs.

General Categories of Treatment Programs

Research studies on addiction treatment typically have classified programs into several general types or modalities. Treatment approaches and individual programs continue to evolve and diversify, and many programs today do not fit neatly into traditional drug addiction treatment classifications. Examples of specific research-based treatment components are described on pages 30–35.

Detoxification and Medically Managed Withdrawal
Detoxification is the process by which the body clears itself of drugs and is often accompanied by unpleasant and sometimes even fatal side effects caused by withdrawal. As stated previously, detoxification alone does not address the psychological, social, and behavioral problems associated with addiction and therefore does not typically produce lasting behavioral changes necessary for recovery.

The process of detoxification often is managed with medications that are administered by a physician in an inpatient or outpatient setting; therefore, it is referred to as "medically managed withdrawal." Detoxification is generally considered a precursor to or a first stage of treatment because it is designed to manage the acute and potentially dangerous physiological effects of stopping drug use. Medications are available to assist in the withdrawal from opioids, benzodiazepines, alcohol, nicotine, barbiturates, and other sedatives. Detoxification should be followed by a formal assessment and referral to subsequent drug addiction treatment.

Further Reading
Kleber, H.D. Outpatient detoxification from opiates. *Primary Psychiatry* 1:42–52, 1996.

Long-Term Residential Treatment

Long-term residential treatment provides care 24 hours a day, generally in nonhospital settings. The best-known residential treatment model is the therapeutic community (TC), with planned lengths of stay between 6 and 12 months. TCs focus on the "resocialization" of the individual and use the program's entire community— including other residents, staff, and the social context— as active components of treatment. Addiction is viewed in the context of an individual's social and psychological deficits, and treatment focuses on developing personal accountability and responsibility as well as socially productive lives. Treatment is highly structured and can be confrontational at times, with activities designed to help residents examine damaging beliefs, self-concepts, and destructive patterns of behavior and adopt new, more harmonious and constructive ways to interact with others. Many TCs offer comprehensive services, which can include employment training and other support services, on site. Research shows that TCs can be modified to treat individuals with special needs, including adolescents, women, homeless individuals, people with severe mental disorders, and individuals in the criminal justice system (see page 35).

Further Reading
Lewis, B.F.; McCusker, J.; Hindin, R.; Frost, R.; and Garfield, F. Four residential drug treatment programs: Project IMPACT. In: J.A. Inciardi, F.M. Tims, and B.W. Fletcher (eds.), *Innovative Approaches in the*

Treatment of Drug Abuse, Westport, CT: Greenwood Press, pp. 45–60, 1993.

Sacks, S.; Banks, S.; McKendrick, K.; and Sacks, J.Y. Modified therapeutic community for co-occurring disorders: A summary of four studies. *Journal of Substance Abuse Treatment* 34(1):112–122, 2008.

Sacks, S.; Sacks, J.; DeLeon, G.; Bernhardt, A.; and Staines, G. Modified therapeutic community for mentally ill chemical "abusers": Background; influences; program description; preliminary findings. Substance Use and Misuse 32(9):1217–1259, 1997.

Stevens, S.J., and Glider, P.J. Therapeutic communities: Substance abuse treatment for women. In: F.M. Tims, G. DeLeon, and N. Jainchill (eds.), Therapeutic Community: *Advances in Research and Application, National Institute on Drug Abuse Research Monograph 144*, NIH Pub. No. 94–3633, U.S. Government Printing Office, pp. 162–180, 1994.

Sullivan, C.J.; McKendrick, K.; Sacks, S.; and Banks, S.M. Modified therapeutic community for offenders with MICA disorders: Substance use outcomes. *American Journal of Drug and Alcohol Abuse* 33(6):823–832, 2007.

Short-Term Residential Treatment

Short-term residential programs provide intensive but relatively brief treatment based on a modified 12-step approach. These programs were originally designed to treat alcohol problems, but during the cocaine epidemic of the mid-1980s, many began to treat other types of substance use disorders. The original residential treatment model consisted of a 3–6-week hospital-based inpatient treatment phase followed by extended outpatient therapy and participation in a self-help group, such as Alcoholics Anonymous. Following stays in residential treatment programs, it is important for individuals to remain engaged in outpatient treatment programs and/or aftercare programs. These programs help to reduce the risk of relapse once a patient leaves the residential setting.

Further Reading

Hubbard, R.L.; Craddock, S.G.; Flynn, P.M.; Anderson, J.; and Etheridge, R.M. Overview of 1-year follow-up outcomes in the Drug Abuse Treatment Outcome Study (DATOS). *Psychology of Addictive Behaviors* 11(4):291–298, 1998.

Miller, M.M. Traditional approaches to the treatment of addiction. In: A.W. Graham and T.K. Schultz (eds.), Principles of Addiction Medicine (2nd ed.). Washington, D.C.: American Society of Addiction Medicine, 1998.

Outpatient Treatment Programs

Outpatient treatment varies in the types and intensity of services offered. Such treatment costs less than residential or inpatient treatment and often is more suitable for people with jobs or extensive social supports. It should be noted, however, that low-intensity programs may offer little more than drug education. Other outpatient models, such as intensive day treatment, can be comparable to residential programs in services and effectiveness, depending on the individual patient's characteristics and needs. In many outpatient programs, group counseling can be a major component. Some outpatient programs are also designed to treat patients with medical or other mental health problems in addition to their drug disorders.

Further Reading

Hubbard, R.L.; Craddock, S.G.; Flynn, P.M.; Anderson, J.; and Etheridge, R.M. Overview of 1-year follow-up outcomes in the Drug Abuse Treatment Outcome Study (DATOS). *Psychology of Addictive Behaviors* 11(4):291–298, 1998.

Institute of Medicine. Treating Drug Problems. Washington, D.C.: National Academy Press, 1990.

McLellan, A.T.; Grisson, G.; Durell, J.; Alterman, A.I.; Brill, P.; and O'Brien, C.P. Substance abuse treatment in the private setting: Are some programs more effective than others? *Journal of Substance Abuse Treatment* 10:243–254, 1993.

Simpson, D.D., and Brown, B.S. Treatment retention and follow-up outcomes in the Drug Abuse Treatment Outcome Study (DATOS). *Psychology of Addictive Behaviors* 11(4):294–307, 1998.

Individualized Drug Counseling

Individualized drug counseling not only focuses on reducing or stopping illicit drug or alcohol use; it also addresses related areas of impaired functioning—such as employment status, illegal activity, and family/social relations—as well as the content and structure of the patient's recovery program. Through its emphasis on short-term behavioral goals, individualized counseling helps the patient develop coping strategies and tools to abstain from drug use and maintain abstinence. The addiction counselor encourages 12-step participation (at least one or two times per week) and makes referrals for needed supplemental medical, psychiatric, employment, and other services.

Group Counseling

Many therapeutic settings use group therapy to capitalize on the social reinforcement offered by peer discussion and to help promote drug-free lifestyles. Research has shown that when group therapy either is offered in conjunction with individualized drug counseling or is formatted to reflect the principles of cognitive-behavioral therapy or contingency management, positive outcomes are achieved. Currently, researchers are testing conditions in which group therapy can be standardized and made more community-friendly.

Further Reading

Crits-Christoph, P.; Gibbons, M.B.; Ring-Kurtz, S.; Gallop, R.; and Present, J. A pilot study of community-friendly manual-guided drug counseling. *Journal of Substance Abuse Treatment;* 2008 Nov. 26; [Epub ahead of print].

Crits-Christoph, P.; Siqueland, L.; Blaine, J.; Frank, A.; Luborsky, L.; Onken, L.S.; et al. Psychosocial treatments for cocaine dependence: National Institute on Drug Abuse Collaborative Cocaine Treatment Study. *Archives of General Psychiatry* 56(6):493–502, 1999.

Treating Criminal Justice–Involved Drug Abusers and Addicted Individuals

Research has shown that combining criminal justice sanctions with drug treatment can be effective in decreasing drug abuse and related crime. Individuals under legal coercion tend to stay in treatment longer and do as well as or better than those not under legal pressure. Often, drug abusers come into contact with the criminal justice system earlier than other health or social systems, presenting opportunities for intervention and treatment prior to, during, after, or in lieu of incarceration—which may ultimately interrupt and shorten a career of drug use. More information on how the criminal justice system can address the problem of drug addiction can be found in *Principles of Drug Abuse Treatment for Criminal Justice Populations: A Research-Based Guide* (National Institute on Drug Abuse, revised 2007).

EVIDENCE-BASED APPROACHES TO DRUG ADDICTION TREATMENT

This section presents several examples of treatment approaches and components that have an evidence base supporting their efficacy. Each approach is designed to address certain aspects of drug addiction and its consequences for the individual, family, and society. Some of the approaches are intended to supplement or enhance existing treatment programs, and others are fairly comprehensive in and of themselves.

The following is not a complete list of efficacious evidence-based treatment approaches. More are under development as part of our continuing support of treatment research.

Pharmadotherapies: Opioid Addiction

Methadone

Methadone maintenance treatment is usually conducted in specialized settings (e.g., methadone maintenance clinics). These specialized treatment programs offer the long-acting synthetic opioid medication methadone at a dosage sufficient to prevent opioid withdrawal, block the effects of illicit opioid use, and decrease opioid craving.

Combined with behavioral treatment: The most effective methadone maintenance programs include individual and/or group counseling, as well as provision of or referral to other needed medical, psychological, and social services. In a study that compared opioid-addicted individuals receiving only methadone to those receiving methadone coupled with counseling, individuals who received only methadone showed some improvement in reducing opioid use; however, the addition of counseling produced significantly more improvement, and the addition of onsite medical/psychiatric, employment, and family services further improved outcomes.

Further Reading

Dole, V.P.; Nyswander, M.; and Kreek, Mj. Narcotic blockade. *Archives of Internal Medicine* 118:304–309, 1996.

McLellan, A.T.; Arndt, I.O.; Metzger, D.; Woody, G.E.; and O'Brien, C.P. The effects of psychosocial services in substance abuse treatment. *JAMA* 269(15):1953–1959, 1993.

Woody, G.E., et al. Psychotherapy for opiate addicts: Does it help? *Archives of General Psychiatry* 40:639–645, 1983.

Buprenorphine

Buprenorphine is a partial agonist (it has both agonist and antagonist properties) at opioid receptors that carries a low risk of overdose. It reduces or eliminates withdrawal symptoms associated with opioid dependence but does not produce the euphoria and sedation caused by heroin or other opioids.

In 2000, Congress passed the Drug Addiction Treatment Act, allowing qualified physicians to prescribe Schedule III, IV, and V medications for the treatment of opioid addiction. This created a major paradigm shift that allowed access to opioid treatment in general medical settings, such as primary care offices, rather than limiting it to specialized treatment clinics.

Buprenorphine was the first medication to be approved under the Drug Addiction Treatment Act and is available in two formulations: Subutex® (a pure form of buprenorphine) and the more commonly prescribed Suboxone® (a combination of buprenorphine and the opioid antagonist naloxone). The unique formulation with naloxone produces severe withdrawal symptoms when addicted individuals inject it to get high, lessening the likelihood of diversion.

Physicians who provide office-based buprenorphine treatment for detoxification and/or maintenance treatment must have special accreditation. These physicians are also required to have the capacity to provide counseling to patients when indicated or, if they do not, to refer patients to those who do.

Office-based treatment of opioid addiction is a cost-effective approach that increases the reach of treatment and the options available to patients. Many patients have life circumstances that make office-based treatment a better option for them than specialty clinics. For example, they may live far away from treatment centers or have working hours incompatible with the clinic hours. Office-based addiction treatment is being offered by primary care physicians, psychiatrists, and other specialists, such as internists and pediatricians.

Patients stabilized on adequate, sustained dosages of methadone or buprenorphine can function normally. They can hold jobs, avoid the crime and violence of the street culture, and reduce their exposure to HIV by stopping or decreasing injection drug use and drug-related high-risk sexual behavior. Patients stabilized on these medications can also engage more readily in counseling and other behavioral interventions essential to recovery and rehabilitation.

> *Patients stabilized on adequate, sustained dosages of methadone or buprenorphine can hold jobs, avoid crime and violence, and reduce their exposure to HIV.*

Further Reading

Fiellin, D.A., et al. Counseling plus buprenorphinenaloxone maintenance therapy for opioid dependence.*The New England Journal of Medicine* 355(4):365–374, 2006.

Fudala P.J., et al. Buprenorphine/Naloxone Collaborative Study Group: Office-based treatment of opiate addiction with a sublingual-tablet formulation of buprenorphine and naloxone. *The New England Journal of Medicine* 349(10):949–958, 2003.

Kosten, T.R., and Fiellin, D.A. U.S. National Buprenorphine Implementation Program: Buprenorphine for office-based practice: Consensus conference overview. *The American Journal on Addictions* 13(Suppl. 1):S1–S7, 2004.

McCance-Katz, E.F. Office-based buprenorphine treatment for opioid-dependent patients. *Harvard Review of Psychiatry* 12(6):321–338, 2004.

Naltrexone

Naltrexone is a long-acting synthetic opioid antagonist with few side effects. An opioid antagonist blocks opioids from binding to their receptors and thereby prevents an addicted individual from feeling the effects associated with opioid use. Naltrexone as a treatment for opioid addiction is usually prescribed in outpatient medical settings, although initiation of the treatment often begins after medical detoxification in a residential setting. To prevent withdrawal symptoms, individuals must be medically detoxified and opioid-free for several days before taking naltrexone. The medication is taken orally either daily or three times a week for a sustained period. When used this way, naltrexone blocks all the effects, including euphoria, of self-administered opioids. The theory behind this treatment is that the repeated absence of the desired effects and the perceived futility of using the opioid will gradually diminish opioid craving and addiction. Naltrexone itself has no subjective effects (that is, a person does not perceive any particular drug effects) or potential for abuse, and it is not addictive. However, patient noncompliance is a common problem. Therefore, a favorable treatment outcome requires an accompanying positive therapeutic relationship, effective counseling or therapy, and careful monitoring of medication compliance. Many experienced clinicians have found naltrexone best suited for highly motivated, recently detoxified patients who desire total abstinence because of external circumstances. Professionals, parolees, probationers, and prisoners in work-release status exemplify this group.

Combined with behavioral treatment: Motivational incentives, such as the offering of prizes or rewards for maintaining abstinence, have been shown to enhance the treatment compliance and efficacy of naltrexone for opioid addiction.

Further Reading

Carroll, K.M., et al. Targeting behavioral therapies to enhance naltrexone treatment of opioid dependence: Efficacy of contingency management and significant other involvement. *Archives of General Psychiatry* 58(8):755–761, 2001.

Cornish, J.W., et al. Naltrexone pharmacotherapy for opioid dependent federal probationers. *Journal of Substance Abuse Treatment* 14(6):529–534, 1997.

Greenstein, R.A.; Arndt, I.C.; McLellan, A.T.; and O'Brien, C.P. Naltrexone: A clinical perspective. *Journal of Clinical Psychiatry* 45(9, Part 2):25–28, 1984.

Preston, K.L.; Silverman, K.; Umbricht, A.; DeJesus, A.; Montoya, I.D.; and Schuster, C.R. Improvement in naltrexone treatment compliance with contingency management. *Drug and Alcohol Dependence* 54(2):127–135, 1999.

Resnick, R.B., and Washton, A.M. Clinical outcome with naltrexone: Predictor variables and followup status in detoxified heroin addicts. *Annals of the New York Academy of Sciences* 311:241–246, 1978.

Tobacco Addiction

Nicotine Replacement Therapy (NRT)

A variety of formulations of nicotine replacement therapies now exist, including the transdermal nicotine patch, nicotine spray, nicotine gum, and nicotine lozenges. Because nicotine is the main addictive ingredient in tobacco, the rationale for NRT is that stable low levels of nicotine will prevent withdrawal symptoms—which often drive continued tobacco use—and help keep people motivated to quit.

Bupropion (Zyban®)

Bupropion was originally marketed as an antidepressant (Wellbutrin®). It has mild stimulant effects through blockade of the reuptake of catecholamines, especially norepinephrine and dopamine. A serendipitous observation among depressed patients was the medication's efficacy in suppressing tobacco craving, promoting cessation without concomitant weight gain. Although bupropion's exact mechanisms of action in facilitating smoking cessation are unclear, it has FDA approval as a smoking cessation treatment.

Varenicline (Chantix®)

Varenicline is the most recently FDA-approved medication for smoking cessation. It acts on a subset of nicotinic receptors (alpha-4 beta-2) thought to be involved in the rewarding effects of nicotine. Varenicline acts as a partial agonist/antagonist at these receptors—this means that it mildly stimulates the nicotine receptor, but not sufficiently to allow the release of dopamine, which is important for the rewarding effects of nicotine. As an antagonist, varenicline also blocks the ability of nicotine to activate dopamine, interfering with the reinforcing effects of smoking, thereby reducing cravings and supporting abstinence from smoking.

Combined with Behavioral Treatment

Each of the above pharmacotherapies is recommended for use in combination with behavioral interventions, including group and individual therapies, as well as telephone quitlines. Through behavioral skills training, patients learn to avoid high-risk situations for smoking relapse and to plan strategies to cope with such situations when necessary. Coping techniques include cigarette refusal skills, assertiveness, and time management skills that patients practice in treatment, social, and work settings. Combined treatment is urged because behavioral and pharmacological treatments are thought to operate by different yet complementary mechanisms that can have additive effects. By dampening craving intensity, medications can give patients a leg up on enacting new strategies and skills.

Further Reading

Alterman, A.I.; Gariti, P.; and Mulvaney, F. Short- and long-term smoking cessation for three levels of intensity of behavioral treatment. *Psychology of Addictive Behaviors* 15:261–264, 2001.

Cinciripini, P.M.; Cinciripini, L.G.; Wallfisch, A.; Haque, W.; and Van Vunakis, H. Behavior therapy and the transdermal nicotine patch: Effects on cessation outcome, affect, and coping. *Journal of Consulting and Clinical Psychology* 64:314–323, 1996.

Hughes, J.R. Combined psychological and nicotine gum treatment for smoking: A critical review. *Journal of Substance Abuse* 3:337–350, 1991.

Jorenby, D.E., et al. Efficacy of varenicline, an á4â2 nicotinic acetylcholine receptor partial agonist, vs placebo or sustained-release bupropion for smoking cessation: A randomized controlled trial. *The Journal of the American Medical Association* 296(1):56–63, 2006.

Stitzer, M. Combined behavioral and pharmacological treatments for smoking cessation. *Nicotine & Tobacco Research* 1:S181–S187, 1999.

Alcohol Addiction

Naltrexone

Naltrexone blocks opioid receptors that are involved in the rewarding effects of drinking and the craving for alcohol. It reduces relapse to heavy drinking, defined as four or more drinks per day for women and five or more for men. Naltrexone cuts relapse risk during the first 3 months by about 36 percent but is less effective in helping patients maintain abstinence.

Acamprosate

Acamprosate (Campral®) acts on the gamma-aminobutyric acid (GABA) and glutamate neurotransmitter systems and is thought to reduce symptoms of protracted withdrawal, such as insomnia, anxiety, restlessness, and dysphoria. Acamprosate has been shown to help dependent drinkers maintain abstinence for several weeks to months, and it may be more effective in patients with severe dependence.

Disulfiram

Disulfiram (Antabuse®) interferes with degradation of alcohol, resulting in the accumulation of acetaldehyde, which, in turn, produces a very unpleasant reaction that includes flushing, nausea, and palpitations if the patient drinks alcohol. The utility and effectiveness of disulfiram are considered limited because compliance is generally poor. However, among patients who are highly motivated, disulfiram can be effective, and some patients use it episodically for high-risk situations, such as social occasions where alcohol is present. It can also be administered in a monitored fashion, such as in a clinic or by a spouse, improving its efficacy.

Topiramate

Topiramate is thought to work by increasing inhibitory (GABA) neurotransmission and reducing stimulatory (glutamate) neurotransmission. Its precise mechanism of action in treating alcohol addiction is not known, and *it has not yet received FDA approval.* Topiramate has been shown in two randomized, controlled trials to significantly improve multiple drinking outcomes, compared with a placebo. Over the course of a 14-week trial, topiramate significantly increased the proportion of patients with 28 consecutive days of abstinence or non-heavy drinking. In both studies, the differences between topiramate and placebo groups were still diverging at the end of the trial, suggesting that the maximum effect may not have yet been reached. Importantly, efficacy was established in volunteers who were drinking upon starting the medication.

Combined with Behavioral Treatment

While a number of behavioral treatments have been shown to be effective in the treatment of alcohol addiction, it does not appear that an additive effect exists between behavioral treatments and pharmacotherapy. Studies have shown that getting help is one of the most important factors in treating alcohol addiction, compared to getting a particular type of treatment.

Further Reading

Anton, R.F.; O'Malley, S.S.; Ciraulo, D.A.; et al., for the COMBINE Study Research Group. Combined pharmacotherapies and behavioral interventions for alcohol dependence: The COMBINE study: A randomized controlled trial. *JAMA* 295(17):2003–2017, 2006.

National Institute on Alcohol Abuse and Alcoholism. *Helping Patients Who Drink Too Much: A Clinician's Guide, Updated 2005 Edition.* Bethesda, MD: NIAAA, updated 2005. Available at *http://www. niaaa.nih.gov /Publications/ducationTrainingMaterials/guide.htm.*

Behavioral Therapies

Behavioral treatments help engage people in drug abuse treatment, provide incentives for them to remain abstinent, modify their attitudes and behaviors related to drug abuse, and increase their life skills to handle stressful circumstances and environmental cues that may trigger intense craving for drugs and prompt another cycle of compulsive abuse. Below are a number of behavioral therapies shown to be effective in addressing substance abuse (effectiveness with particular drugs is denoted in parentheses).

Cognitive-Behavioral Therapy (Alcohol, Marijuana, Cocaine, Methamphetamine, Nicotine)

Cognitive-behavioral therapy was developed as a method to prevent relapse when treating problem drinking, and later was adapted for cocaine-addicted individuals. Cognitive-behavioral strategies are based on the theory that learning processes play a critical role in the development of maladaptive behavioral patterns. Individuals learn to identify and correct problematic behaviors by applying a range of different skills that can be used to stop drug abuse and to address a range of other problems that often co-occur with it.

Cognitive-behavioral therapy generally consists of a collection of strategies intended to enhance self-control. Specific techniques include exploring the positive and negative consequences of continued use, self-monitoring to recognize drug cravings early on and to identify high-risk situations for use, and developing strategies for coping with and avoiding high-risk situations and the desire to use. A central element of this treatment is anticipating likely problems and helping patients develop effective coping strategies.

Research indicates that the skills individuals learn through cognitive-behavioral approaches remain after the completion of treatment. In several studies, most people receiving a cognitive-behavioral approach maintained the gains they made in treatment throughout the following year.

Current research focuses on how to produce even more powerful effects by combining cognitive-behavioral therapy with medications for drug abuse and with other types of behavioral therapies. Researchers are also evaluating how best to train treatment providers to deliver cognitive-behavioral therapy.

Further Reading

Carroll, K., et al. Efficacy of disulfiram and cognitive behavior therapy in cocaine-dependent outpatients: A randomized placebo-controlled trial. *Archives of General Psychiatry* 61(3):264–272, 2004.

Carroll, K.; Rounsaville, B.; and Keller, D. Relapse prevention strategies for the treatment of cocaine abuse. *American Journal of Drug and Alcohol Abuse* 17(3):249–265, 1991.

Carroll, K.; Rounsaville, B.; Nich, C.; Gordon, L.; Wirtz, P.; and Gawin, F. One-year follow-up of psychotherapy and pharmacotherapy for cocaine dependence: Delayed emergence of psychotherapy effects. *Archives of General Psychiatry* 51(12):989–997, 1994.

Carroll, K.; Sholomskas, D.; Syracuse, G.; Ball, S.A.; Nuro, K.; and Fenton, L.R. We don't train in vain: A dissemination trial of three strategies of training clinicians in cognitive-behavioral therapy. *Journal of Consulting and Clinical Psychology* 73(1):106–115, 2005.

Carroll, K.M., et al. The use of contingency management and motivational/skills-building therapy to treat young adults with marijuana dependence. *Journal of Consulting and Clinical Psychology* 74(5):955–966, 2006.

Community Reinforcement Approach Plus Vouchers *(Alcohol, Cocaine)*

Community Reinforcement Approach (CRA) Plus Vouchers is an intensive 24-week outpatient therapy for treatment of cocaine and alcohol addiction. The treatment goals are twofold:

- To maintain abstinence long enough for patients to learn new life skills to help sustain it
- To reduce alcohol consumption for patients whose drinking is associated with cocaine use

Patients attend one or two individual counseling sessions each week, where they focus on improving family relations, learning a variety of skills to minimize drug use, receiving vocational counseling, and developing new recreational activities and social networks. Those who also abuse alcohol receive clinic-monitored disulfiram (Antabuse) therapy. Patients submit urine samples two or three times each week and receive vouchers for cocaine-negative samples. The value of the vouchers increases with consecutive clean samples. Patients may exchange vouchers for retail goods that are consistent with a cocaine-free lifestyle.

This approach facilitates patients' engagement in treatment and systematically aids them in gaining substantial periods of cocaine abstinence. The approach has been tested in urban and rural areas and used successfully in outpatient treatment of opioid-addicted adults and with inner-city methadone maintenance patients with high rates of intravenous cocaine abuse.

Further Reading

Higgins, S.T., et al. Community reinforcement therapy for cocaine-dependent outpatients. *Archives of General Psychiatry* 60(10):1043–1052, 2003.

Roozen, H.G.; Boulogne, Jj.; van Tulder, M.W.; van den Brink, W.; De Jong, C.Aj.; and Kerhof, J.F.M. A systemic review of the effectiveness of the community reinforcement approach in alcohol, cocaine and opioid addiction. *Drug and Alcohol Dependence* 74(1):1–13, 2004.

Silverman, K., et al. Sustained cocaine abstinence in methadone maintenance patients through voucher-based reinforcement therapy. *Archives of General Psychiatry* 53(5):409–415, 1996.

Smith, J.E.; Meyers, Rj.; and Delaney, H.D. The community reinforcement approach with homeless alcohol-dependent individuals. *Journal of Consulting and Clinical Psychology* 66(3):541–548, 1998.

Stahler, Gj., et al. Development and initial demonstration of a community-based intervention for homeless, cocaine-using, African-American women. *Journal of Substance Abuse Treatment* 28(2):171–179, 2005.

Contingency Management Interventions/Motivational Incentives (Alcohol, Stimulants, Opioids, Marijuana, Nicotine)

Research has demonstrated the effectiveness of treatment approaches using contingency management principles, which involve giving patients in drug treatment the chance to earn low-cost incentives in exchange for drug-free urine samples. These incentives include prizes given immediately or vouchers exchangeable for food items, movie passes, and other personal goods. Studies conducted in both methadone programs and psychosocial counseling treatment programs demonstrate that incentive-based interventions are highly effective in increasing treatment retention and promoting abstinence from drugs.

Some concerns have been raised that a prize-based contingency management intervention could promote gambling—as it contains an element of chance—and that pathological gambling and substance use disorders can be comorbid. However, studies have shown no differences in gambling over time between those assigned to the contingency management conditions and those in the usual care groups, indicating that this prize-based contingency management procedure did not promote gambling behavior.

Further Reading

Budney, Aj.; Moore, B.A.; Rocha, H.L.; and Higgins, S.T. Clinical trial of abstinence-based vouchers and cognitive-behavioral therapy for cannabis dependence. *Journal of Consulting and Clinical Psychology* 74(2):307–316, 2006.

Budney, Aj.; Roffman, R.; Stephens, R.S.; and Walker, D. Marijuana dependence and its treatment. *Addiction Science & Clinical Practice* 4(1):4–16, 2007.

Elkashef, A.; Vocci, F.; Huestis, M.; Haney, M.; Budney, A.; Gruber, A.; and el-Guebaly, N. Marijuana neurobiology and treatment. *Substance Abuse* 29(3):17–29, 2008.

Peirce, J.M., et al. Effects of lower-cost incentives on stimulant abstinence in methadone maintenance treatment: A National Drug Abuse Treatment Clinical Trials Network study. *Archives of General Psychiatry* 63(2):201–208, 2006.

Petry, N.M., et al. Effect of prize-based incentives on outcomes in stimulant abusers in outpatient psychosocial treatment programs: A National Drug Abuse Treatment Clinical Trials Network study. *Archives of General Psychiatry* 62(10):1148–1156, 2005.

Petry, N.M., et al. Prize-based contingency management does not increase gambling. *Drug and Alcohol Dependence* 83(3):269–273, 2006.

Prendergast, M.; Podus, D.; Finney, J.; Greenwell, L.; and Roll, J. Contingency management for treatment of substance use disorders: A meta-analysis. *Addiction* 101(11):1546–1560, 2006.

Roll, J.M., et al. Contingency management for the treatment of methamphetamine use disorders. *The American Journal of Psychiatry* 163(11):1993–1999, 2006.

Motivational Enhancement Therapy
(*Alcohol, Marijuana, Nicotine*)

Motivational Enhancement Therapy (MET) is a patient-centered counseling approach for initiating behavior change by helping individuals resolve ambivalence about engaging in treatment and stopping drug use. This approach employs strategies to evoke rapid and internally motivated change, rather than guiding people stepwise through the recovery process. This therapy consists of an initial assessment battery session, followed by two to four individual treatment sessions with a therapist. In the first treatment session, the therapist provides feedback to the initial assessment battery, stimulating discussion about personal substance use and eliciting self-motivational statements. Motivational interviewing principles are used to strengthen motivation and build a plan for change. Coping strategies for high-risk situations are suggested and discussed with the patient. In subsequent sessions, the therapist monitors change, reviews cessation strategies being used, and continues to encourage commitment to change or sustained abstinence. Patients sometimes are encouraged to bring a significant other to sessions.

Research on MET suggests that its effects depend on the type of drug used by participants and on the goal of the intervention. This approach has been used successfully with alcoholics to improve both treatment engagement and treatment outcomes (e.g., reductions in problem drinking). MET has also been used successfully with adult marijuana-dependent individuals in combination with cognitive-behavioral therapy, comprising a more comprehensive treatment approach. The results of MET are mixed for participants abusing other drugs (e.g., heroin, cocaine, nicotine, etc.) and for adolescents who tend to use multiple drugs. In general, MET seems to be more effective for engaging drug abusers in treatment than for producing changes in drug use.

Further Reading

Baker, A., et al. Evaluation of a motivational interview for substance use with psychiatric in-patient services. *Addiction* 97(10):1329–1337, 2002.

Haug, N.A.; Svikis, D.S.; and Diclemente, C. Motivational enhancement therapy for nicotine dependence in methadone-maintained pregnant women. *Psychology of Addictive Behaviors* 18(3):289–292, 2004.

Marijuana Treatment Project Research Group. Brief treatments for cannabis dependence: Findings from a randomized multisite trial. *Journal of Consulting and Clinical Psychology* 72(3):455–466, 2004.

Miller, W.R.; Yahne, C.E.; and Tonigan, J.S. Motivational interviewing in drug abuse services: A randomized trial. *Journal of Consulting and Clinical Psychology* 71(4):754–763, 2003.

Stotts, A.L.; Diclemente, C.C.; and Dolan-Mullen, P. One-to-one: A motivational intervention for resistant pregnant smokers. *Addictive Behaviors* 27(2):275–292, 2002.

The Matrix Model *(Stimulants)*

The Matrix Model provides a framework for engaging stimulant (e.g., methamphetamine and cocaine) abusers in treatment and helping them achieve abstinence. Patients learn about issues critical to addiction and relapse, receive direction and support from a trained therapist, become familiar with self-help programs, and are monitored for drug use through urine testing.

The therapist functions simultaneously as teacher and coach, fostering a positive, encouraging relationship with the patient and using that relationship to reinforce positive behavior change. The interaction between the therapist and the patient is authentic and direct but not confrontational or parental. Therapists are trained to conduct treatment sessions in a way that promotes the patient's self-esteem, dignity, and self-worth. A positive relationship between patient and therapist is critical to patient retention.

Treatment materials draw heavily on other tested treatment approaches and, thus, include elements of relapse prevention, family and group therapies, drug education, and self-help participation. Detailed treatment manuals contain worksheets for individual sessions; other components include family education groups, early recovery skills groups, relapse prevention groups, combined sessions, urine tests, 12-step programs, relapse analysis, and social support groups.

A number of studies have demonstrated that participants treated using the Matrix Model show statistically significant reductions in drug and alcohol use, improvements in psychological indicators, and reduced risky sexual behaviors associated with HIV transmission.

Further Reading
Huber, A.; Ling, W.; Shoptaw, S.; Gulati, V.; Brethen, P.; and Rawson, R. Integrating treatments for methamphetamine abuse: A psychosocial perspective. *Journal of Addictive Diseases* 16(4):41–50, 1997.

Rawson, R., et al. An intensive outpatient approach for cocaine abuse: The Matrix model. *Journal of Substance Abuse Treatment* 12(2):117–127, 1995.

Rawson, R.A., et al. A comparison of contingency management and cognitive-behavioral approaches during methadone maintenance treatment for cocaine dependence. *Archives of General Psychiatry* 59(9):817–824, 2002.

✳12-Step Facilitation Therapy (*Alcohol, Stimulants, Opiates*)

Twelve-step facilitation therapy is an active engagement strategy designed to increase the likelihood of a substance abuser becoming affiliated with and actively involved in 12-step self-help groups and, thus, promote abstinence. Three key aspects predominate: acceptance, which includes the realization that drug addiction is a chronic, progressive disease over which one has no control, that life has become unmanageable because of drugs, that willpower alone is insufficient to overcome the problem, and that abstinence is the only alternative; surrender, which involves giving oneself over to a higher power, accepting the fellowship and support structure of other recovering addicted individuals, and following the recovery activities laid out by the 12-step program; and active involvement in 12-step meetings and related activities. While the efficacy of 12-step programs (and 12-step facilitation) in treating alcohol dependence has been established, the research on other abused drugs is more preliminary but promising for helping drug abusers sustain recovery. NIDA has recognized the need for more research in this area and is currently funding a community-based study to examine the impact of 12-step facilitation therapy for methamphetamine and cocaine abusers.

Further Reading
Carroll, K.M.; Nich, C.; Ball, S.A.; McCance, E.; Frankforter, T.L.; and Rounsaville, Bj. One-year follow-up of disulfiram and psychotherapy for cocaine-alcohol users: Sustained effects of treatment. *Addiction* 95(9):1335–1349, 2000.

Donovan D.M., and Wells E.A. "Tweaking 12-step": The potential role of 12-Step self-help group involvement in methamphetamine recovery. *Addiction* 102(Suppl. 1):121–129, 2007.

Project MATCH Research Group. Matching alcoholism treatments to client heterogeneity: Project MATCH posttreatment drinking outcomes. *Journal of Studies on Alcohol* 58(1)7–29, 1997.

Behavioral Couples Therapy

Behavioral Couples Therapy (BCT) is a therapy for drug abusers with partners. BCT uses a sobriety/abstinence contract and behavioral principles to reinforce abstinence from drugs and alcohol. It has been studied as an add-on to individual and group therapy and typically involves 12 weekly couple sessions, lasting approximately 60 minutes each. Many studies support BCT's efficacy with alcoholic men and their spouses; four studies support its efficacy with drug-abusing men and women and their significant others. BCT also has been shown to produce higher treatment attendance, naltrexone adherence, and rates of abstinence than individual treatment, along with fewer drug-related, legal, and family problems at 1-year followup.

Recent research has focused on making BCT more community-friendly by adapting the therapy for delivery in fewer sessions and in a group format. Research is also being done to demonstrate cost-effectiveness and to test therapy effectiveness according to therapist training.

Further Reading

Fals-Stewart, W.; Klosterman, K.; Yates, B.T.; O'Farrell, T.J.; and Birchler, G.R. Brief relationship therapy for alcoholism: A randomized clinical trial examining clinical efficacy and cost-effectiveness. *Psychology of Addictive Behaviors* 19(4):363–371, 2005.

Fals-Stewart, W.; O'Farrell, T.J.; and Birchler, G.R. Behavioral couples therapy for male methadone maintenance patients: Effects on drug-using behavior and relationship adjustment. *Behavior Therapy* 32(2):391–411, 2001.

Kelley, M. L., and Fals-Stewart, W. Couples- versus individual-based therapy for alcohol and drug abuse: Effects on children's psychosocial functioning. *Journal of Consulting and Clinical Psychology* 70(2):417–427, 2002.

Klostermann, K.; Fals-Stewart, W.; and Yates, B.T. Behavioral couples therapy for substance abuse: A cost analysis. *Alcoholism: Clinical Experimental Research* 28(Suppl.):164A, 2004.

Winters, J.; Fals-Stewart, W.; O'Farrell, T.J.; Birchler, G.R; and Kelley, M.L.
Behavioral couples therapy for female substance-abusing patients: Effects
on substance use and relationship adjustment. *Journal of Consulting and
Clinical Psychology* 70(2):344–355, 2002.

Behavioral Treatments for Adolescents

Drug-abusing and addicted adolescents have unique treatment needs.
Research has shown that treatments designed for and tested in adult
populations often need to be modified to be effective in adolescents. Family
involvement is a particularly important component for interventions targeting
youth. Below are examples of behavioral interventions that employ these
principles and have shown efficacy for treating addiction in youth.

Multisystemic Therapy

Multisystemic Therapy (MST) addresses the factors associated with
serious antisocial behavior in children and adolescents who abuse alcohol and
other drugs. These factors include characteristics of the child or adolescent
(e.g., favorable attitudes toward drug use), the family (poor discipline, family
conflict, parental drug abuse), peers (positive attitudes toward drug use),
school (dropout, poor performance), and neighborhood (criminal subculture).
By participating in intensive treatment in natural environments (homes,
schools, and neighborhood settings), most youths and families complete a full
course of treatment. MST significantly reduces adolescent drug use during
treatment and for at least 6 months after treatment. Fewer incarcerations and
out-of-home juvenile placements offset the cost of providing this intensive
service and maintaining the clinicians' low caseloads.

Further Reading

Henggeler, S.W.; Clingempeel, W.G.; Brondino, Mj.; and Pickrel, S.G. Four-
year follow-up of multisystemic therapy with substance-abusing and
substance-dependent juvenile offenders. *Journal of the American
Academy of Child and Adolescent Psychiatry* 41(7):868–874, 2002.
Henggeler, S.W., et al. Home-based multisystemic therapy as an alternative to
the hospitalization of youths in psychiatric crisis: Clinical outcomes.
Journal of the American Academy of Child and Adolescent Psychiatry
38(11):1331–1339, 1999.

Henggeler, S.W.; Halliday-Boykins, C.A.; Cunningham, P.B.; Randall, J.; Shapiro, S.B.; and Chapman, J.E. Juvenile drug court: Enhancing outcomes by integrating evidence-based treatments. *Journal of Consulting and Clinical Psychology* 74(1):42–54, 2006.

Henggeler, S.W.; Pickrel, S.G.; Brondino, Mj.; and Crouch, J.L. Eliminating (almost) treatment dropout of substance-abusing or dependent delinquents through home-based multisystemic therapy. *The American Journal of Psychiatry* 153(3):427–428, 1996.

Huey, Sj.; Henggeler, S.W.; Brondino, Mj.; and Pickrel, S.G. Mechanisms of change in multisystemic therapy: Reducing delinquent behavior through therapist adherence and improved family functioning. *Journal of Consulting and Clinical Psychology* 68(3):451–467, 2000.

Multidimensional Family Therapy for Adolescents

Multidimensional Family Therapy (MDFT) for adolescents is an outpatient family-based alcohol and other drug abuse treatment for teenagers. MDFT views adolescent drug use in terms of a network of influences (individual, family, peer, community) and suggests that reducing unwanted behavior and increasing desirable behavior occur in multiple ways in different settings. Treatment includes individual and family sessions held in the clinic, in the home, or with family members at the family court, school, or other community locations.

During individual sessions, the therapist and adolescent work on important developmental tasks, such as developing decisionmaking, negotiation, and problemsolving skills. Teenagers acquire vocational skills and skills in communicating their thoughts and feelings to deal better with life stressors. Parallel sessions are held with family members. Parents examine their particular parenting styles, learning to distinguish influence from control and to have a positive and developmentally appropriate influence on their children.

Further Reading

Dennis, M., et al. The Cannabis Youth Treatment (CYT) Study: Main findings from two randomized clinical trials. *Journal of Substance Abuse Treatment* 27(3):197–213, 2004.

Liddle, H.A.; Dakof, G.A.; Parker, K.; Diamond, G.S.; Barrett, K;, and Tejeda, M. Multidimensional family therapy for adolescent drug abuse: Results of a randomized clinical trial. *The American Journal of Drug and Alcohol Abuse* 27(4):651–688, 2001.

Liddle, H.A., and Hogue, A. Multidimensional family therapy for adolescent substance abuse. In E.F. Wagner and H.B. Waldron (eds.), *Innovations in Adolescent Substance Abuse Interventions*. London: Pergamon/Elsevier Science, pp. 227–261, 2001.

Liddle, H.A.; Rowe, C.L.; Dakof, G.A.; Ungaro, R.A.; and Henderson, C.E. Early intervention for adolescent substance abuse: Pretreatment to posttreatment outcomes of a randomized clinical trial comparing multidimensional family therapy and peer group treatment. *Journal of Psychoactive Drugs* 36(1):49–63, 2004.

Schmidt, S.E.; Liddle, H.A.; and Dakof, G.A. Effects of multidimensional family therapy: Relationship of changes in parenting practices to symptom reduction in adolescent substance abuse. *Journal of Family Psychology* 10(1):1–16, 1996.

Brief Strategic Family Therapy

Brief Strategic Family Therapy (BSFT) targets family interactions that are thought to maintain or exacerbate adolescent drug abuse and other co-occurring problem behaviors. Such problem behaviors include conduct problems at home and at school, oppositional behavior, delinquency, associating with antisocial peers, aggressive and violent behavior, and risky sexual behavior. BSFT is based on a family systems approach to treatment, where family members' behaviors are assumed to be interdependent such that the symptoms of any one member (the drug-abusing adolescent, for example) are indicative, at least in part, of what else is going on in the family system. The role of the BSFT counselor is to identify the patterns of family interaction that are associated with the adolescent's behavior problems and to assist in changing those problem-maintaining family patterns. BSFT is meant to be a flexible approach that can be adapted to a broad range of family situations in various settings (mental health clinics, drug abuse treatment programs, other social service settings, and families' homes) and in various treatment modalities (as a primary outpatient intervention, in combination with residential or day treatment, and as an aftercare/continuing-care service to residential treatment).

Further Reading

Coatsworth, J.D.; Santisteban, D.A.; McBride, C.K.; and Szapocznik, J. Brief Strategic Family Therapy versus community control: Engagement, retention, and an exploration of the moderating role of adolescent severity. *Family Process* 40(3):313–332, 2001.

Santisteban, D.A.; Coatsworth, J.D.; Perez-Vidal, A.; Mitrani, V.; Jean-Gilles, M.; and Szapocznik, J. Brief Structural/Strategic Family Therapy with African-American and Hispanic high-risk youth. *Journal of Community Psychology* 25(5):453–471, 1997.

Santisteban, D.A.; Suarez-Morales, L.; Robbins, M.S.; and Szapocznik, J. Brief strategic family therapy: Lessons learned in efficacy research and challenges to blending research and practice. *Family Process* 45(2):259–271, 2006.

Santisteban, D.A.; Szapocznik, J.; Perez-Vidal, A.; Kurtines, W.M.; Murray, Ej.; and Laperriere, A. Efficacy of intervention for engaging youth and families into treatment and some variables that may contribute to differential effectiveness. *Journal of Family Psychology* 10(1):35–44, 1996.

Szapocznik, J., et al. Engaging adolescent drug abusers and their families in treatment: A strategic structural systems approach. *Journal of Consulting and Clinical Psychology* 56(4):552–557, 1988.

RESOURCES

General Inquiries

Inquiries about NIDA's behavioral treatment research activities should be directed to the Division of Clinical Neuroscience and Behavioral Research at 301-443-0107. For questions regarding NIDA's medications development program, please contact the Division of Pharmacotherapies and Medical Consequences of Drug Abuse at 301-443-6173. For questions regarding treatment organization, management, financing, effectiveness, and cost-effectiveness research, please contact the Division of Epidemiology, Services and Prevention Research at 301-443-4060; for questions regarding NIDA-supported clinical trials, please call the National Drug Abuse Treatment Clinical Trials Network at 301-443-6697; and for questions regarding NIDA's HIV/AIDS research, please contact the AIDS Research Program at 301-443-1470. Additional general information is available at www.drugabuse.gov or by calling 301-443-1124.

National Institute on Alcohol Abuse and Alcoholism (NIAAA)

NIAAA provides leadership in the national effort to reduce alcohol-related problems by conducting and supporting research in a wide range of scientific areas, including genetics, neuroscience, epidemiology, health risks and benefits of alcohol consumption, prevention, and treatment; coordinating and collaborating with other research institutes and Federal programs on alcohol-related issues; collaborating with international, national, State, and local institutions, organizations, agencies, and programs engaged in alcohol-related work; and translating and disseminating research findings to health care providers, researchers, policymakers, and the public. Additional information is available at www.niaaa.nih.gov or by calling 301-443-3860.

National Institute of Mental Health (NIMH)

The mission of NIMH is to transform the understanding and treatment of mental illnesses through basic and clinical research, paving the way for prevention, recovery, and cure. In support of this mission, NIMH generates research and promotes research training to fulfill the following four objectives: promote discovery in the brain and behavioral sciences to fuel research on the causes of mental disorders; chart mental illness trajectories to determine when, where, and how to intervene; develop new and better interventions that incorporate the diverse needs and circumstances of people with mental illnesses; and strengthen the public health impact of NIMHsupported research. Additional information is available at www.nimh.nih.gov or by calling 301-443-4513.

Center for Substance Abuse Treatment (CSAT)

CSAT, a part of the Substance Abuse and Mental Health Services Administration (SAMHSA), is responsible for supporting treatment services through a block grant program, as well as disseminating findings to the field and promoting their adoption. CSAT also operates the 24-hour National Treatment Referral Hotline (1-800-662-HELP), which offers information and referral services to people seeking treatment programs and other assistance. CSAT publications are available through the National Clearinghouse on Alcohol and Drug Information (1-800-729-6686). Additional information about CSAT can be found on SAMHSA's Web site at www.csat.samhsa.gov.

Selected NIDA Educational Resources on Drug Addiction Treatment

The following are available from the NIDA DrugPubs Research Dissemination Center, the National Technical Information Service (NTIS), or the Government Printing Office (GPO). To order, refer to the DrugPubs (877-NIDANIH [643-2644]), NTIS (1-800-553-6847), or GPO (202-512-1800) number provided with the resource description.

Manuals and Clinical Reports
Principles of Drug Abuse Treatment for Criminal Justice Populations: A Research-Based Guide (Revised 2007). Provides 13 essential treatment principles and includes resource information and answers to frequently asked questions. Publication #NIH 07-5316. Available online at *www.nida.nih.gov/PODAT_CJ*.

Measuring and Improving Cost, Cost-Effectiveness, and Cost-Benefit for Substance Abuse Treatment Programs (1999). Offers tools for substance abuse treatment program managers to calculate the costs of their programs and investigate the relationship between those costs and treatment outcomes. Available online at *www.nida.nih.gov/IMPCOST/IMPCOSTIndex.html*.

A Cognitive-Behavioral Approach: Treating
Cocaine Addiction (1998). This is the first in NIDA's "Therapy Manuals for Drug Addiction" series. Describes cognitive-behavioral therapy, a short-term, focused approach to helping cocaine-addicted individuals become abstinent from cocaine and other drugs. Available online at *www.nida.nih.gov/TXManuals/CBT/CBT1.html*.

A Community Reinforcement Plus Vouchers Approach: Treating Cocaine Addiction (1998). This is the second in NIDA's "Therapy Manuals for Drug Addiction" series. This treatment integrates a community reinforcement approach with an incentive program that uses vouchers. Available online at *www.nida.nih.gov/ TXManuals/CRA/CRA1.html*.

An Individual Drug Counseling Approach to Treat Cocaine Addiction: The Collaborative Cocaine Treatment Study Model (1999). This is the third in NIDA's "Therapy Manuals for Drug Addiction" series. Describes specific behavioral/cognitive models that can be implemented in a wide range of drug abuse treatment settings. Available online at *www.nida.nih.gov/ TXManuals/IDCA/IDCA1.html*.

Addiction Severity Index (ASI). Provides a structured clinical interview designed to collect information about substance use and functioning in life areas from adult clients seeking drug abuse treatment. For more information on using the ASI and to obtain copies of the most recent edition, please visit *www.tresearch.org/resources/instruments.htm#top*.

Other Useful Publications

A Collection of NIDA Notes Articles That Address Drug Abuse Treatment (Reprinted 2008). This collection of NIDA Notes articles showcases NIDA treatment-related research. Publication #NN0026. Available online at www.nida.nih.gov/NIDA_Notes/NN0026.html.

Alcohol Alert (published by NIAAA). This is a quarterly bulletin that disseminates important research findings on alcohol abuse and alcoholism. Available online at www.niaaa.nih.gov/Publications/AlcoholAlerts.

Drugs, Brains, and Behavior: The Science of Addiction (Reprinted 2008). This publication provides an overview of the science behind the disease of addiction. Publication #NIH 08–5605. Available online at www.nida. nih.gov/scienceofaddiction.

NIAAA Clinical Guidelines/Related Resources. This Web site has information to help clinicians in the screening, diagnosis, and treatment of patients who drink too much. Available online at www.niaaa.nih.gov/ Publications/EducationTrainingMaterials/guide.htm.

NIDA InfoFacts: Treatment Approaches for Drug Addiction (Revised 2008). This is a fact sheet covering research findings on effective treatment approaches for drug abuse and addiction. Available online at www.nida.nih. gov/ infofacts/treatmeth.html.

Research Report Series: Therapeutic Community (2002). This report provides information on the role of residential drug-free settings and their role in the treatment process. Publication #PHD947. Available online at www.nida.nih.gov/ResearchReports/Therapeutic/default.html.

The NIDA Clinical Toolbox: Science-Based Materials for Drug Abuse Treatment Providers (2000). This Web site contains science-based materials for drug abuse treatment providers. Links are provided to treatment manuals, Research Reports, and more. Available online at www.nida.nih.gov/TB/Clinical/ClinicalToolbox.html.

Initiatives Designed to Move Treatment Research into Practice

Clinical Trials Network

Assessing the real-world effectiveness of evidence-based treatments is a crucial step in bringing research to practice.

Established in 1999, NIDA's National Drug Abuse Treatment Clinical Trials Network (CTN) uses community settings with diverse patient populations and conditions to adjust and test protocols to meet the practical needs of addiction treatment. Since its inception, the CTN has tested pharmacological and behavioral interventions for drug abuse and addiction, along with common co-occurring conditions (e.g. HIV and PTSD) among various target populations, including adolescent drug abusers, pregnant drug-abusing women, and Spanish-speaking patients. The CTN has also tested prevention strategies in drug-abusing groups at high risk for hepatitis C (HCV) and HIV and has become a key element of NIDA's multipronged approach to move promising science-based drug addiction treatments rapidly into community settings. For more information on the CTN, please visit *www.drugabuse.gov/CTN/Index.htm.*

Criminal Justice–Drug Abuse Treatment Studies

NIDA is taking an approach similar to the CTN to enhance treatment for drug-addicted individuals involved with the criminal justice system through the CJ-DATS (Criminal Justice–Drug Abuse Treatment Studies). Whereas NIDA's CTN has as its overriding mission the improvement of the quality of drug abuse treatment by moving innovative approaches into the larger community, research supported through CJ-DATS is designed to effect change by bringing new treatment models into the criminal justice system and thereby improve outcomes for offenders with substance use disorders. It seeks to achieve better integration of drug abuse treatment with other public health and public safety forums and represents a collaboration among NIDA; the Substance Abuse and Mental Health Services Administration (SAMHSA); the Centers for Disease Control and Prevention (CDC); Department of Justice agencies; and a host of drug treatment, criminal justice, and health and social service professionals.

Blending Teams

Another way in which NIDA is seeking to actively move science into practice is through a joint venture with SAMHSA and its nationwide network of Addiction Technology Transfer Centers (ATTCs). This process involves the collaborative efforts of community treatment practitioners, SAMHSA trainers, and NIDA researchers, some of whom form "Blending Teams" to create products and devise strategic dissemination plans for them. Through the creation of products designed to foster adoption of new treatment strategies, Blending Teams are instrumental in getting the latest evidence-based tools and practices into the hands of treatment professionals. To date, a number of products have been completed.

Topics have included increasing awareness of the value of buprenorphine therapy and enhancing healthcare workers' proficiency in using tools such as the Addiction Severity Index (ASI), motivational interviewing, and motivational incentives. For more information on Blending products, please visit NIDA's Web site at *www.nida.nih.gov/blending.*

Other Federal Resources

NIDA DrugPubs Research Dissemination Center. NIDA publications and treatment materials are available from this information source. Staff provide assistance in English and Spanish, and have TDD capability. Phone: 877-NIDA-NIH (877-643-2644); TTY/TDD: 240-645-0228; fax: 240-645-0227; e-mail: drugpubs@nida.nih.gov; Web site: *www.drugabuse.gov.*

The National Registry of Evidence-Based Programs and Practices. This database of interventions for the prevention and treatment of mental and substance use disorders is maintained by SAMHSA and can be accessed at *www.nrepp.samhsa.gov.*

The National Clearinghouse for Alcohol and Drug Information (NCADI). Publications from other Federal agencies are available from this information source. Staff provide assistance in English and Spanish, and have TDD capability. Phone: 800-729-6686; Web site: *www.ncadi.samhsa.gov.*

The National Institute of Justice (NIJ). As the research agency of the Department of Justice, NIJ supports research, evaluation, and demonstration programs relating to drug abuse in the context of crime and the criminal justice system. For information, including a wealth of publications, contact the National Criminal Justice Reference Service at 800-851-3420 or 301-519-5500; or visit *www.ojp.usdoj.gov/nij.*

Clinical Trials. For more information on federally and privately supported clinical trials please visit *www.clinicaltrials.gov.*

ACKNOWLEDGMENTS

The National Institute on Drug Abuse wishes to thank the following individuals for reviewing this publication.

Martin W. Adler, Ph.D.

Temple University School of Medicine

Andrea G. Barthwell, M.D.

Encounter Medical Group

Kathleen Brady, M.D., Ph.D.

Medical University of South Carolina

Greg Brigham, Ph.D. Maryhaven

Lawrence S. Brown, Jr., M.D., M.P. H. Addiction Research and

Treatment Corporation

James F. Callahan, D.P.A. American Society of

Addiction Medicine

Kathleen M. Carroll, Ph.D.

Yale University School of Medicine

H. Westley Clark, M.D., J.D.,

M.P.H., CAS, FASAM

Center for Substance Abuse Treatment

Richard R. Clayton, Ph.D. University of Kentucky

Linda B. Cottler, Ph.D. Washington University School of Medicine

David P. Friedman, Ph.D.

Bowman Gray School of Medicine

NIH Publication No. 09–4180

Printed October 1999; Reprinted July 2000, February 2008; Revised April 2009.

In: Drug Addiction: Science and Treatment   ISBN: 978-1-61470-004-3
Editors: N. Jacobs and L. C. Dubois   © 2012 Nova Science Publishers, Inc.

Chapter 3

PRINCIPLES OF DRUG ABUSE TREATMENT FOR CRIMINAL JUSTICE POPULATIONS[*]

National Institute on Drug Abuse

1. DRUG ADDICTION IS A BRAIN DISEASE THAT AFFECTS BEHAVIOR

Drug addiction has well-recognized cognitive, behavioral, and physiological characteristics that contribute to continued use of drugs despite the harmful consequences. Scientists have also found that chronic drug abuse alters the brain's anatomy and chemistry and that these changes can last for months or years after the individual has stopped using drugs. This transformation may help explain why addicts are at a high risk of relapse to drug abuse even after long periods of abstinence and why they persist in seeking drugs despite deleterious consequences.

---

[*] This is an edited, reformatted and augmented version of a National Institute on Drug Abuse publication, dated September 2006, Revised September 2007.

2. RECOVERY FROM DRUG ADDICTION REQUIRES EFFECTIVE TREATMENT, FOLLOWED BY MANAGEMENT OF THE PROBLEM OVER TIME

Drug addiction is a serious problem that can be treated and managed throughout its course. Effective drug abuse treatment engages participants in a therapeutic process, retains them in treatment for an appropriate length of time, and helps them learn to maintain abstinence over time. Multiple episodes of treatment may be required. Outcomes for drug abusing offenders in the community can be improved by monitoring drug use and by encouraging continued participation in treatment.

3. TREATMENT MUST LAST LONG ENOUGH TO PRODUCE STABLE BEHAVIORAL CHANGES

In treatment, the drug abuser is taught to break old patterns of thinking and behaving and to learn new skills for avoiding drug use and criminal behavior. Individuals with severe drug problems and co-occurring disorders typically need longer treatment (e.g., a minimum of 3 months) and more comprehensive services. Early in treatment, the drug abuser begins a therapeutic process of change. In later stages, he or she addresses other problems related to drug abuse and learns how to manage the problem.

4. ASSESSMENT IS THE FIRST STEP IN TREATMENT

A history of drug or alcohol use may suggest the need to conduct a comprehensive assessment to determine the nature and extent of an individual's drug problems, establish whether problems exist in other areas that may affect recovery, and enable the formulation of an appropriate treatment plan. Personality disorders and other mental health problems are prevalent in offender populations; therefore, comprehensive assessments should include mental health evaluations with treatment planning for these problems.

5. TAILORING SERVICES TO FIT THE NEEDS OF THE INDIVIDUAL IS AN IMPORTANT PART OF EFFECTIVE DRUG ABUSE TREATMENT FOR CRIMINAL JUSTICE POPULATION

Individuals differ in terms of age, gender, ethnicity and culture, problem severity, recovery stage, and level of supervision needed. Individuals also respond differently to different treatment approaches and treatment providers. In general, drug treatment should address issues of motivation, problemsolving, and skill-building for resisting drug use and criminal behavior. Lessons aimed at supplanting drug use and criminal activities with constructive activities and at understanding the consequences of one's behavior are also important to include. Treatment interventions can facilitate the development of healthy interpersonal relationships and improve the participant's ability to interact with family, peers, and others in the community.

6. DRUG USE DURING TREATMENT SHOULD BE CAREFULLY MONITORED

Individuals trying to recover from drug addiction may experience a relapse, or return, to drug use. Triggers for drug relapse are varied; common ones include mental stress and associations with peers and social situations linked to drug use. An undetected relapse can progress to serious drug abuse, but detected use can present opportunities for therapeutic intervention. Monitoring drug use through urinalysis or other objective methods, as part of treatment or criminal justice supervision, provides a basis for assessing and providing feedback on the participant's treatment progress. It also provides opportunities to intervene to change unconstructive behavior—determining rewards and sanctions to facilitate change, and modifying treatment plans according to progress.

7. TREATMENT SHOULD TARGET FACTORS THAT ARE ASSOCIATED WITH CRIMINAL BEHAVIOR

"Criminal thinking" is a combination of attitudes and beliefs that support a criminal lifestyle and criminal behavior. These can include feeling entitled to have things one's own way, feeling that one's criminal behavior is justified, failing to be responsible for one's actions, and consistently failing to anticipate or appreciate the consequences of one's behavior. This pattern of thinking often contributes to drug use and criminal behavior. Treatment that provides specific cognitive skills training to help individuals recognize errors in judgment that lead to drug abuse and criminal behavior may improve outcomes.

8. CRIMINAL JUSTICE SUPERVISION SHOULD INCORPORATE TREATMENT PLANNING FOR DRUG ABUSING OFFENDERS, AND TREATMENT PROVIDERS SHOULD BE AWARE OF CORRECTIONAL SUPERVISION REQUIREMENTS

The coordination of drug abuse treatment with correctional planning can encourage participation in drug abuse treatment and can help treatment providers incorporate correctional requirements as treatment goals. Treatment providers should collaborate with criminal justice staff to evaluate each individual's treatment plan and ensure that it meets correctional supervision requirements, as well as that person's changing needs, which may include housing and childcare; medical, psychiatric, and social support services; and vocational and employment assistance. For offenders with drug abuse problems, planning should incorporate the transition to community-based treatment and links to appropriate postrelease services to improve the success of drug treatment and re-entry. Abstinence requirements may necessitate a rapid clinical response, such as more counseling, targeted intervention, or increased medication, to prevent relapse. Ongoing coordination between treatment providers and courts or parole and probation officers is important in addressing the complex needs of these re-entering individuals.

9. Continuity of Care Is Essential for Drug Abusers Re-Entering the Community

Those who complete prison-based treatment and continue with treatment in the community have the best outcomes. Continuing drug abuse treatment helps the recently released offender deal with problems that become relevant only at re-entry, such as learning to handle situations that could lead to relapse, learning how to live drug-free in the community, and developing a drug-free peer support network. Treatment in prison or jail can begin a process of therapeutic change, resulting in reduced drug use and criminal behavior postincarceration. Continuing drug treatment in the community is essential to sustaining these gains.

10. A Balance of Rewards and Sanctions Encourages Prosocial Behavior and Treatment Participation

When providing correctional supervision of individuals participating in drug abuse treatment, it is important to reinforce positive behavior. Nonmonetary "social reinforcers" such as recognition for progress or sincere effort can be effective, as can graduated sanctions that are consistent, predictable, and clear responses to noncompliant behavior. Generally, less punitive responses are used for early and less serious noncompliance, with increasingly severe sanctions issuing from continued problem behavior. Rewards and sanctions are most likely to have the desired effect when they are perceived as fair and when they swiftly follow the targeted behavior.

11. Offenders with Co-Occurring Drug Abuse and Mental Health Problems Often Require an Integrated Treatment Approach

High rates of mental health problems are found both in offender populations and in those with substance abuse problems. Drug abuse treatment can sometimes address depression, anxiety, and other mental health problems. Personality, cognitive, and other serious mental disorders can be difficult to treat and may disrupt drug treatment. The presence of co-occurring disorders may require an integrated approach that combines drug abuse treatment with psychiatric treatment, including the use of medication. Individuals with either a substance abuse or mental health problem should be assessed for the presence of the other.

12. Medications Are an Important Part of Treatment for Many Drug Abusing Offenders

Medicines such as methadone and buprenorphine for heroin addiction have been shown to help normalize brain function and should be made available to individuals who could benefit from them. Effective use of medications can also be instrumental in enabling people with co-occurring mental health problems to function successfully in society. Behavioral strategies can increase adherence to medication regimens.

13. Treatment Planning for Drug Abusing Offenders who Are Living in or Re-Entering the Community Should Include Strategies to Prevent and Treat Serious, Chronic Medical Conditions, Such as HIV/AIDS, Hepatitis B and C, and Tuberculosis

The rates of infectious diseases, such as hepatitis, tuberculosis, and HIV/AIDS, are higher in drug abusers, incarcerated offenders, and offenders under community supervision than in the general population. Infectious diseases affect not just the offender, but also the criminal justice system and the wider community. Consistent with Federal and State laws, drug-involved offenders should be offered testing for infectious diseases and receive counseling on their health status and on ways to modify risk behaviors. Probation and parole officers who monitor offenders with serious medical conditions should link them with appropriate healthcare services, encourage compliance with medical treatment, and re-establish their eligibility for public health services (e.g., Medicaid, county health departments) before release from prison or jail.

PREFACE

From the time it was established in 1974, the National Institute on Drug Abuse (NIDA) has supported research on drug abuse treatment for people involved with the criminal justice system.

Findings show unequivocally that providing comprehensive drug abuse treatment to criminal offenders works, reducing both drug abuse and criminal recidivism. Given the swelling prison population, attributable in large part to drug-related offenses accompanied by high rates of recidivism, it is a matter of public health and safety to make drug abuse treatment a key component of the criminal justice system. Indeed, addressing the treatment needs of substance abusing offenders is critical to reducing overall crime and other drug-related societal burdens, such as lost job productivity.

Scientific research shows that drug abuse treatment can work even when an individual enters it under legal mandate. However, only a small percentage of those who need treatment actually receive it, and often the treatment provided is not sufficient. To be effective, treatment must begin in prison and be sustained after release through participation in community treatment programs. By engaging in a continuing therapeutic process, people can learn how to avoid relapse and withdraw from a life of crime.

As reflected in our collaborative Criminal Justice–Drug Abuse Treatment Studies (CJ–DATS) Initiative, NIDA is committed to working across organizational boundaries to improve substance abuse treatment services. Multiple studies from different scientific disciplines have helped us understand the basic neurobiology of addiction, along with what constitutes effective treatment to help individuals recover. Increased understanding of the complex biological, behavioral, and social consequences of addiction helps to strengthen behavioral and medical interventions aimed at motivating and sustaining abstinence.

This booklet—a complement to NIDA's Principles of Drug Addiction Treatment: A Research-Based Guide—is intended to describe the treatment principles and research findings that have particular relevance to the criminal justice community and to treatment professionals working with drug abusing offenders. It is divided into three main sections: (1) research findings on addicted offenders distilled into 13 essential principles (see pages 1–5), (2) a series of frequently asked questions (FAQs) about drug abuse treatment for those involved with the criminal justice system, and (3) a resource section that provides Web sites for additional information. A summary of the research underlying both the principles and the FAQs is available on NIDA's Web site at www.drugabuse.gov.

With the release of this landmark publication's revised edition, we are optimistic that correctional agencies are starting to realize how implementing drug treatment programs can help achieve public health and safety goals for the Nation.

Nora D. Volkow, M.D.
Director
National Institute on Drug Abuse

INTRODUCTION

The Connection between Drug Abuse and Crime Is Well Known

Drug abuse is implicated in at least three types of drug-related offenses: (1) offenses defined by drug possession or sales, (2) offenses directly related to drug abuse (e.g., stealing to get money for drugs), and (3) offenses related to a lifestyle that predisposes the drug abuser to engage in illegal activity, for example, through association with other offenders or with illicit markets. Individuals who use illicit drugs are more likely to commit crimes, and it is common for many offenses, including violent crimes, to be committed by individuals who had used drugs or alcohol prior to committing the crime, or who were using at the time of the offense.

After a nationally representative survey of State correctional agencies was conducted in 2005, Criminal Justice–Drug Abuse Treatment Studies (CJ–DATS) investigators estimated that nearly 8 million adults are involved in the justice system (Taxman, Young, Wiersema, et al., 2007). Almost 5 million individuals are on probation or under parole supervision (Glaze and Bonczar, 2006; Taxman, Young, Wiersema, et al., 2007), with drug law violators accounting for the largest percentage of these parolees. The substance abuse or dependence rates of offenders are more than four times that of the general population (National Institute of Justice, 2003; U.S. Department of Health and Human Services, 2006). In a 2004 survey, the Bureau of Justice Statistics (BJS) estimated that about 53 percent of State and 45 percent of Federal prisoners met Diagnostic and Statistical Manual for Mental Disorders (DSM) criteria for drug abuse or dependence (Mumola and Karberg, 2006). Of those surveyed, 14.8 percent of State and 17.4 percent of Federal prisoners reported having received drug treatment since admission (Mumola and Karberg, 2006). Juvenile justice systems also report high levels of drug abuse. A survey of juvenile detainees in 2000 found that about 56 percent of the boys and 40 percent of the girls tested positive for drug use at the time of their arrest (National Institute of Justice, 2003).

Although the past several decades have witnessed an increased interest in providing substance abuse treatment services for criminal justice offenders, only a small percentage of offenders has access to adequate services, especially in jails and community correctional facilities (Taxman, Perdoni, and Harrison, 2007). Not only is there a gap in the availability of these services for offenders, but often there are few choices in the types of services provided.

Treatment that is of insufficient quality and intensity or that is not well suited to the needs of offenders may not yield meaningful reductions in drug use and recidivism. Untreated substance abusing offenders are more likely than treated offenders to relapse to drug abuse and return to criminal behavior. This can bring about re-arrest and re-incarceration, jeopardizing public health and public safety and taxing criminal justice system resources. Treatment offers the best alternative for interrupting the drug abuse/criminal justice cycle for offenders with drug abuse problems.

Drug abuse treatment can be incorporated into criminal justice settings in a variety of ways. These include treatment as a condition of probation, drug courts that blend judicial monitoring and sanctions with treatment, treatment in prison followed by community-based treatment after release, and treatment under parole or probation supervision. Drug abuse treatment can benefit from the cross-agency coordination and collaboration of criminal justice professionals, substance abuse treatment providers, and other social service agencies. By working together, the criminal justice and treatment systems can optimize resources to benefit the health, safety, and well-being of the individuals and communities they serve.

Treatment offers the best alternative for interrupting the drug abuse/criminal justice cycle.

FREQUENTLY ASKED QUESTIONS (FAQs)

1. Why Do People Involved in the Criminal Justice System Continue Abusing Drugs?

The answer to this perplexing question spans basic neurobiological, psychological, social, and environmental factors. The repeated use of addictive drugs eventually changes how the brain functions. Resulting brain changes, which accompany the transition from voluntary to compulsive drug use, affect the brain's natural inhibition and reward centers, causing the addict to use drugs in spite of the adverse health, social, and legal consequences (Volkow, Fowler, Wang, et al., 1993; Volkow, Hitzemann, Wang, et al., 1992; Volkow and Li, 2004). Craving for drugs may be triggered by contact with the people, places, and things associated with prior drug use, as well as by stress.

Forced abstinence without treatment does not cure addiction. Abstinent individuals must still learn how to avoid relapse, including those who have been incarcerated and may have been abstinent for a long period of time.

Addictive drugs cause long-lasting changes in the brain

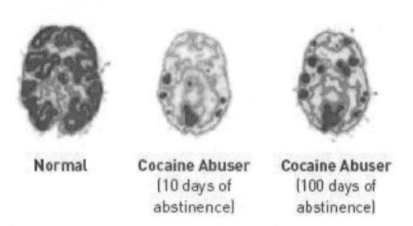

Source: Volkow et al, 1992, 1993.

PET scans showing glucose metabolism in healthy brain and cocaine-addicted brains. Even after 100 days of abstinence, glucose metabolism has not returned to normal levels.

Potential risk factors for released offenders include pressures from peers and even family members to return to drug use and a criminal lifestyle. Tensions of daily life—violent associates, few opportuni-ties for legitimate employment, lack of safe housing, even the need to comply with correctional supervision conditions—can also create stressful situations that can precipitate a relapse to drug use.

Research on how the brain is affected by drug abuse promises to help us learn much more about the mechanics of drug-induced brain changes and their relationship to addiction. Research also reveals that with effective drug abuse treatment, individuals can overcome persistent drug effects and lead healthy, productive lives.

2. Why Should Drug Abuse Treatment Be Provided to Offenders?

The case for treating drug abusing offenders is compelling. Drug abuse treatment improves outcomes for drug abusing offenders and has beneficial effects for public health and safety. Effective treatment decreases future drug use and drug-related criminal behavior, can improve the individual's relationships with his or her family, and may improve prospects for employment.

Outcomes for substance abusing individuals can be improved when criminal justice personnel work in tandem with treatment providers on drug abuse treatment needs and supervision requirements. Treatment needs that can be assessed after arrest include substance abuse severity, mental health problems, and physical health. Defense attorneys, prosecutors, and judges need to work together during the prosecution and sentencing phases of the criminal justice process to determine suitable treatment programs that meet the offender's needs. Through drug courts, diversion programs, pretrial release programs conditional on treatment, and conditional probation with sanctions, the offender can participate in community-based drug abuse treatment while under criminal justice supervision. In some instances, the judge may recommend that the offender participate in treatment while serving jail or prison time or require it as part of continuing correctional supervision postrelease.

3. How Effective is Drug Abuse Treatment for Criminal Justice-Involved Individuals?

Treatment is an effective intervention for drug abusers, including those who are involved with the criminal justice system. However, the effectiveness of drug treatment depends on both the individual and the program, and on whether interventions and treatment services are available and appropriate for the individual's needs. To amend attitudes, beliefs, and behaviors that support drug use, the drug abuser must engage in a therapeutic change process. Longitudinal outcome studies find that those who participate in community-based drug abuse treatment programs commit fewer crimes than those who do not participate.

4. Are All Drug Abusers in the Criminal Justice System Good Candidates for Treatment?

A history of drug use does not in itself indicate the need for drug abuse treatment. Offenders who meet drug dependence criteria should be given higher priority for treatment than those who do not. Less intensive interventions, such as drug abuse education or self-help participation, may be appropriate for those not meeting criteria for drug dependence. Services such as family-based interventions for juveniles, psychiatric treatment, or cognitive-behavioral "criminal thinking" interventions may be a higher priority for some offenders, and individuals with mental health problems may require specialized services (see FAQ Nos. 6 and 12).

Low motivation to participate in treatment or to end drug abuse should not preclude access to treatment if other criteria are met. Motivational enhancement interventions may be useful in these cases. Examples include motivational interviewing and contingency management techniques, which often provide tangible rewards in exchange for meeting program goals. Legal pressure that encourages abstinence and treatment participation may also help these individuals by improving retention and catalyzing longer treatment stays.

Drug abuse treatment is also effective for offenders who have a history of serious and violent crime, particularly if they receive intensive, targeted services. The economic benefits in avoided crime and costs to crime victims (e.g., medical costs, lost earnings, and loss in quality of life) may be substantial for these high-risk offenders. Treating them requires a high degree of coordination between drug abuse treatment providers and criminal justice personnel to ensure that treatment and criminogenic needs are appropriately addressed.

> *Outcomes can be improved when criminal justice personnel work in tandem with treatment providers.*

5. Is Legally Mandated Treatment Effective?

Often the criminal justice system can apply legal pressure to encourage offenders to participate in drug abuse treatment; or treatment can be mandated, for example, through a drug court or as a condition of pretrial release, probation, or parole.

A large percentage of those admitted to drug abuse treatment cite legal pressure as an important reason for seeking treatment.

Most studies suggest that outcomes for those who are legally pressured to enter treatment are as good as or better than outcomes for those who entered treatment without legal pressure. Those under legal pressure also tend to have higher attendance rates and to remain in treatment for longer periods, which can also have a positive impact on treatment outcomes.

> *Legal pressure can increase treatment attendance and improve retention.*

6. Are Relapse Risk Factors Different in Offender Populations? How Should Drug Abuse Treatment Deal with these Risk Factors?

Often, drug abusing offenders have problems in other areas. Examples include family difficulties, limited social skills, educational and employment problems, mental health disorders, infectious diseases, and other medical problems. Treatment should take these problems into account, because they can increase the risk of drug relapse and criminal recidivism if left unaddressed.

Stress is often a contributing factor to relapse, and offenders who are re-entering society face many challenges and stressors, including reuniting with family members, securing housing, and complying with criminal justice supervision requirements. Even the many daily decisions that most people face can be stressful for those recently released from a highly controlled prison environment.

Other threats to recovery include a loss of support from family or friends, which incarcerated people may experience. Drug abusers returning to the community may also encounter family, friends, or associates still involved in drugs or crime and be enticed to resume a criminal and drug using lifestyle.

Returning to environments or activities associated with prior drug use may trigger strong cravings and cause a relapse. A coordinated approach by treatment and criminal justice staff provides the best way to detect and intervene with these and other threats to recovery. In any case, treatment is needed to provide the skills necessary to avoid or cope with situations that could lead to relapse.

Treatment staff should identify the offender's unique relapse risk factors and periodically re-assess and modify the treatment plan as needed. Generally, continuing or re-emerging drug use during treatment requires a clinical response—either increasing the "dosage" or level of treatment, or changing the treatment intervention.

> *Returning to environments associated with drug use may trigger cravings and cause a relapse.*

7. What Treatment and other Health Services Should Be Provided to Drug Abusers Involved with the Criminal Justice System?

One of the goals of treatment planning is to match evidence-based interventions to individual needs at each stage of drug treatment. Over time, various combinations of treatment services may be required. Evidence-based interventions include cognitive-behavioral therapy to help participants learn positive social and coping skills, contingency management approaches to reinforce positive behavioral change, and motivational enhancement to increase treatment engagement and retention. In those addicted to opioid drugs, agonist/partial agonist medications can also help normalize brain function, and antagonist medications can facilitate abstinence. For juvenile offenders, treatments that involve the family and other aspects of the drug abuser's environment have established efficacy.

Drug abuse treatment plans for incarcerated offenders can anticipate their eventual re-entry into the community by incorporating relevant transition plans and services. Drug abusers often have mental and physical health, family counseling, parenting, educational, and vocational needs, so medical, psychological, and social services are often crucial components of successful treatment. Case management approaches can be used to provide assistance in obtaining drug abuse treatment and community services.

8. How Long Should Drug Abuse Treatment Last for Individuals Involved in the Criminal Justice System?

While individuals progress through drug abuse treatment at different rates, one of the most reliable findings in treatment research is that lasting reductions in criminal activity and drug abuse are related to length of treatment. Generally, better outcomes are associated with treatment that lasts longer than 90 days, with the greatest reductions in drug abuse and criminal behavior accruing to those who complete treatment. Again, legal pressure can improve retention rates.

A longer continuum of treatment may be indicated for individuals with severe or multiple problems.

Research has shown that participation in a prison-based therapeutic community followed by community-based treatment after release can reduce the risk of recidivism to criminal behavior as well as relapse to drug use.

Early phases of treatment help the participant stop using drugs and begin a therapeutic process of change. Later stages address other problems related to drug abuse and, importantly, help the individual learn how to self-manage the drug problem.

Because addiction is a chronic disease, drug relapse and return to treatment are common features of an individual's path to recovery, so treatment may need to extend over a long period of time and across multiple episodes of care. It is also the case that those with the most severe problems can participate in treatment and achieve positive outcomes.

Treatment in the criminal justice system reduces drug abuse and recidivism

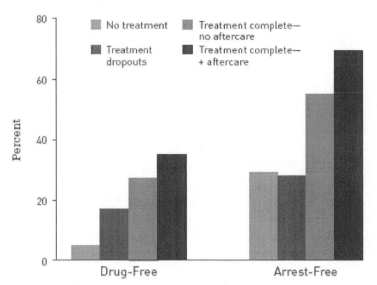

Source: Martin, et al., 1999.

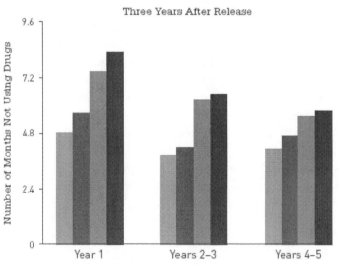

Source: Butzin, et al., 2005.

9. How Can Rewards and Sanctions Be Used Effectively with Drug-Involved Offenders in Treatment?

The systematic application of behavioral management principles underlying reward and punishment can help individuals reduce their drug use and criminal behavior. Rewards and sanctions are most likely to change behavior when they are certain to follow the targeted behavior, when they follow swiftly, and when they are perceived as fair.

It is important to recognize and reinforce progress toward responsible, abstinent behavior. Rewarding positive behavior is more effective in producing long-term positive change than punishing negative behavior. Nonmonetary rewards such as social recognition can be as effective as monetary rewards. A graduated range of rewards given for meeting predetermined goals can be an effective strategy. In community-based treatment, contingency management strategies use voucher-based incentives or rewards, such as bus tokens, to reinforce abstinence (measured by negative drug tests) or to shape progress toward other treatment goals, such as program session attendance or compliance with medication regimens. Contingency management is most effective when the contingent reward closely follows the behavior being monitored.

Graduated sanctions, which invoke less punitive responses for early and less serious noncompliance and increasingly severe sanctions for more serious or continuing problems, can be an effective tool in conjunction with drug testing. The effective use of graduated sanctions involves consistent, predictable, and clear responses to noncompliant behavior.

Drug testing can determine when an individual is having difficulties with recovery. The first response to drug use detected through urinalysis should be clinical—for example, an increase in treatment intensity or a change to an alternative treatment. This often requires coordination between the criminal justice staff and the treatment provider. (Note that more intensive treatment should not be considered a sanction, but rather a routine progression in healthcare practice when a treatment appears less effective than expected.)

Behavioral contracting can employ both rewards and sanctions.

A behavioral contract is an explicit agreement between the participant and the treatment provider or criminal justice monitor (or among all three) that specifies proscribed behaviors and associated sanctions, as well as positive goals and rewards for success. Behavioral contracting can instill a sense of procedural justice because both the necessary steps toward progress and the sanctions for violating the contract are specified and understood in advance.

> *It is important to recognize and reinforce progress toward responsible, abstinent behavior*

10. What Is the Role of Medications in Treating Substance Abusing Offenders?

Medications can be an important component of effective drug abuse treatment for offenders. By allowing the body to function normally, they enable the addict to leave behind a life of crime and drug abuse. For example, opioid agonist/partial agonist medications, which act at the same receptors as heroin, morphine, and natural brain chemicals (endorphins), tend to be well tolerated and can help an individual remain in treatment. Antagonist medications, which work by blocking the effects of a drug, are effective but often are not taken as prescribed. Despite evidence of their effectiveness, addiction medications are underutilized in the treatment of drug abusers within the criminal justice system. Still, some jurisdictions have found ways to successfully implement medication therapy for drug abusing offenders.

Effective medications have been developed for opiates/heroin and alcohol:

- *Opiates/Heroin.* Long-term opiate abuse results in a desensitization of the brain's opiate receptors to endorphins, the body's natural opioids. Methadone acts on the same receptors as the natural endorphins, stabilizing the craving that otherwise results in compulsive use of heroin or other illicit opiates. Methadone is effective in reducing opiate use, drug-related criminal behavior, and HIV risk behavior. Buprenorphine is a partial agonist and acts on the same receptors as morphine (a full agonist), but without producing the same level of dependence or withdrawal symptoms. Suboxone® is a unique formulation of buprenorphine that contains naloxone, an opioid antagonist, which limits diversion by causing severe withdrawal symptoms in those who inject it to get "high," but has no adverse effects when taken orally, as prescribed. Naltrexone, an opiate antagonist, blocks the effects of opiates.
- *Alcohol.* Disulfiram (also known as Antabuse) is an aversion therapy that induces nausea if alcohol is consumed. Acamprosate works by restoring normal balance to the brain's glutamate neurotransmitter system, helping to reduce alcohol craving. Naltrexone, which blocks

some of alcohol's pleasurable effects, is also approved by the Food and Drug Administration (FDA) for treatment of alcohol abuse.

Medications can be an important component of effective addiction treatment for offenders.

11. How Can the Criminal Justice and Drug Abuse Treatment Systems Reduce the Spread of HIV/AIDS, Hepatitis, and other Infectious Diseases among Drug Abusing Offenders?

It is critical for the criminal justice and drug abuse treatment systems to be involved in efforts to reduce the spread of HIV/AIDS and other infectious diseases, which occur at higher rates among drug abusers in the criminal justice system than among the general population. The prevalence of AIDS has been estimated to be approximately five times higher among incarcerated offenders than in the general population. In addition, individuals in the criminal justice system represent a significant portion of hepatitis B, hepatitis C, and tuberculosis cases in the United States. Although most infectious diseases are contracted in the community and not in correctional settings, they must be treated in the correctional setting once diagnosed.

Infectious diseases among offenders who are re-entering or living within the community present a serious public health challenge. While incarcerated, offenders often have access to adequate healthcare, which offers opportunities for integrating strategies to address medical, mental health, and drug abuse problems. Offenders with infectious diseases who are returning to their communities should be linked with community-based medical care prior to release. Community health, drug treatment, and criminal justice agencies should work together to offer education, screening, counseling, prevention, and treatment programs for HIV/AIDS, hepatitis, and other infectious diseases to offenders in or returning to the community. Drug abuse treatment can decrease the spread of infectious disease by reducing high-risk behaviors such as needle sharing and unprotected sex.

The need to negotiate access to health services and adhere to complex treatment protocols places a large burden on the addicted offender, and many offenders fall through the cracks. Untreated or deteriorating medical or mental health problems increase the risk of relapse to drug abuse and to possible re-arrest and re-incarceration.

> *The prevalence of AIDS is five times higher among incarcerated offenders than the general population.*

12. What Works for Offenders with Co-Occurring Substance Abuse and Mental Disorders?

It is important to adequately assess mental disorders and to address them as part of effective drug abuse treatment. Many types of co-occurring mental health problems can be successfully addressed in standard drug abuse treatment programs. However, individuals with serious mental disorders may require an integrated treatment approach designed for treating patients with co-occurring mental health problems and substance use disorders. Although not readily available, specialized therapeutic community "MICA" (for "mentally ill chemical abuser") programs are promising for patients with co-occurring mental and addictive problems.

Much progress has been made in developing effective medications for treating mental disorders, including a number of antidepressants, antianxiety agents, mood stabilizers, and antipsychotics. These medications may be critical for treatment success with offenders who have co-occurring mental disorders such as depression, anxiety disorders, bipolar disorder, or schizophrenia. Cognitive-behavioral therapy can be effective for treating some mental health problems, particularly when combined with medications. Contingency management can improve adherence to medications, and intensive case management may be useful for linking severely mentally ill individuals with drug abuse treatment, mental health care, and community services.

13. Is Providing Drug Abuse Treatment to Offenders Worth the Financial Investment?

In 2002, it was estimated that the cost to society of drug abuse was $180.9 billion (Office of National Drug Control Policy [ONDCP], 2004), a substantial portion of which—$107.8 billion—is associated with drug-related crime, including criminal justice system costs and costs borne by victims of crime. The cost of treating drug abuse (including research, training, and prevention efforts) was estimated to be $15.8 billion, a fraction of these overall societal costs (ONDCP, 2004).

Drug abuse treatment is cost effective in reducing drug use and bringing about associated healthcare, crime, and incarceration cost savings. Positive net economic benefits are consistently found for drug abuse treatment across various settings and populations. The largest economic benefit of treatment is seen in avoided costs of crime (incarceration and victimization costs), with greater economic benefits resulting from treating offenders with co-occurring mental health problems and substance use disorders. Residential prison treatment is more cost effective if offenders attend treatment postrelease, according to research (Martin, Butzin, Saum, and Inciardi, 1999). Drug courts also convey positive economic benefits, including participant-earned wages and avoided incarceration and future crime costs.

> *The largest economic benefit of treatment is seen in avoided costs of crime.*

14. What Are the Unique Treatment Needs for Women in the Criminal Justice System?

Although women are incarcerated at far lower rates than men, the number and percentage of incarcerated women have grown substantially in recent years. Between 1995 and 2005, the number of men in prisons and jails grew by about a third, while the number of incarcerated women more than doubled (Harrison and Beck, 2006). Women in prison are likely to have a different set of problems and needs than men, presenting particular treatment challenges. For example, incarcerated women in treatment are significantly more likely than incarcerated men to have severe substance abuse histories, as well as co-occurring physical health and psychological problems (Messina, Burdon, Hagopian, and Prendergast, 2006). Approximately 50 percent of female offenders are likely to have histories of physical or sexual abuse. Women are also more likely than men to be victims of domestic violence. Past or current victimization can contribute to drug or alcohol abuse, depression, post-traumatic stress disorder, and criminal activity.

Incarcerated women have high rates of substance abuse, mental disorders, and other health problems

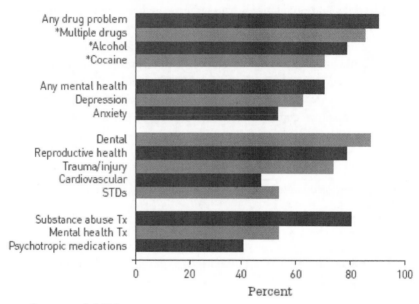

Source: Staton, at al, 2003.
* Note: Graph shows lifetime percentages except for multiple drugs, alcohol, and cocaine, which are the percent reporting use in the 30 days prior to incarceration. (N=60).

Treatment programs serving both men and women can provide effective treatment for their female clients. However, gender-specific programs may be more effective for female offenders, particularly those with histories of trauma and abuse. Female offenders are more likely to need medical and mental health services, childcare services, and assistance in finding housing and employment. Following a comprehensive assessment, women with mental health disorders should receive appropriate treatment and case management, including victim services as needed. For female offenders with children, parental responsibilities can conflict with their ability to participate in drug treatment. Regaining or retaining custody of their children can also motivate mothers to participate in treatment. Treatment programs may improve retention by offering childcare services and parenting classes.

15. What Are the Unique Treatment Needs of Juveniles in the Criminal Justice System?

In recent years, there has been a dramatic increase in the number of juveniles with substance abuse problems involved in the criminal and juvenile justice systems. From 1986 to 1996, drug-related juvenile incarcerations increased nearly threefold. In 2002, about 60 percent of detained boys and nearly half of the girls tested positive for drug use. The number of juvenile court cases involving drug offenses more than doubled between 1993 and 1998, and 116,781 adolescents under the age of 18 were arrested for drug violations in 2002. One study found that about one-half of both male and female juvenile detainees met criteria for a substance use disorder (Teplin, Abram, McClelland, et al., 2002).

Juveniles entering the criminal justice system can bring a number of serious issues with them—substance abuse, academic failure, emotional disturbances, physical health issues, family problems, and a history of physical or sexual abuse. Girls make up nearly one-third of juvenile arrests, a high percentage reporting some form of emotional, physical, or sexual abuse. Effectively addressing these issues requires their gaining access to comprehensive assessment, treatment, case management, and support services appropriate for their age and developmental stage. Assessment is particularly important, because not all adolescents who have used drugs need treatment. For those who do, there are several points in the juvenile justice continuum where treatment has been integrated, including juvenile drug courts, community-based supervision, juvenile detention, and community re-entry.

Families play an important role in the recovery of substance abusing juveniles, but this influence can be either positive or negative. Parental substance abuse or criminal involvement, physical or sexual abuse by family members, and lack of parental involvement or supervision are all risk factors for adolescent substance abuse and delinquent behavior. Thus, the effective treatment of juvenile substance abusers often requires a family-based treatment model that targets family functioning and the increased involvement of family members. Effective adolescent treatment approaches include multisystemic therapy, multidimensional family therapy, and functional family therapy. These interventions show promise in strengthening families and decreasing juvenile substance abuse and delinquent behavior.

> *Effective treatment of juvenile substance abusers often requires a family-based treatment model.*

RESOURCES

Many resources are available on the Internet. The following are useful links:

General Information

NIDA Web site: www.drugabuse.gov.
General Inquires: NIDA Public Information Office 301-443–1124

Federal Resources

Bureau of Justice Assistance (BJA) Substance Abuse Programs
www.ojp.usdoj.gov/bja/ programs/substance_abu.html.

Bureau of Justice Statistics (BJS) Statistics on Drugs and Crime
www.ojp.usdoj.gov/bjs/ drugs.htm.

Center for Substance Abuse Treatment (CSAT) Substance Abuse and Mental Health Services Administration (SAMHSA)
www.csat.samhsa.gov.

Federal Bureau of Prisons (BOP) Substance Abuse Treatment
www.bop.gov/inmate programs/substance.jsp.

National Criminal Justice Reference Service (NCJRS)
www.ncjrs.gov.

National Institute on Alcohol Abuse and Alcoholism (NIAAA)
www.niaaa.nih.gov.

National Institute of Corrections (NIC)
www.nicic.org.
National Institute of Justice (NIJ)
www.ojp.usdoj.gov/nij

National Institute of Mental Health (NIMH)
www.nimh.nih.gov.

Office of Applied Studies (OAS) Substance Abuse and Mental Health
Services Administration (SAMHSA)
www.oas.samhsa.gov

Office of Justice Programs (OJP)
www.ojp.usdoj.gov.

Office of Juvenile Justice and Delinquency Prevention (OJJDP)
www.ojjdp.ncjrs.org.

ACKNOWLEDGMENTS

NIDA wishes to thank the following individuals for their guidance and
comments during the development and review of this publication:

Steven Belenko, Ph.D.
Center on Evidence-based Interventions for Crime and Addiction
Treatment Research Institute

Peter J. Delany, Ph.D.
Division of Treatment and Recovery Research National Institute on
Alcohol Abuse and Alcoholism

Richard Dembo, Ph.D.
Department of Criminology University of South Florida

Gary D. Field, Ph.D. (Retired)
Mental Health Alignment Work Group Oregon Department of Corrections

Kevin Knight, Ph.D.
Institute of Behavioral Research Texas Christian University

Douglas Longshore, Ph.D.
UCLA Integrated Substance Abuse Programs

Roger H. Peters, Ph.D.
Department of Mental Health Law and Policy
Florida Mental Health Institute University of South Florida

This publication was written by Bennett W. Fletcher, Ph.D., and Redonna K. Chandler, Ph.D., National Institute on Drug Abuse. Additional guidance and editing were provided by Jack B. Stein, Ph.D., and the Office of Science Policy and Communications.

REFERENCES

Butzin, C.A.; Martin, S.S.; and Inciardi, J.A. Treatment during transition from prison to community and subsequent illicit drug use. *Journal of Substance Abuse Treatment* 28(4):351–358, 2005.

Glaze, L.E. and Bonczar, T.P. *Probation and parole in the United States, 2005.* Washington, DC: U.S. Department of Justice, Office of Justice Programs, Bureau of Justice Statistics, 2006.

Harrison, P.M. and Beck, A.J. *Prisoners in 2005.* Washington, DC: U.S. Department of Justice, Office of Justice Programs, Bureau of Justice Statistics, 2006.

Martin, S.S.; Butzin, C.A.; Saum, C.A; and Inciardi, J.A. Three-year outcomes of therapeutic community treatment for drug-involved offenders in Delaware: from prison to work release to aftercare. *The Prison Journal* 79(3):294–320, 1999.

Messina, N.; Burdon, W.; Hagopian, G.; and Prendergast, M. Predictors of prison-based treatment outcomes: a comparison of men and women participants. *The American Journal of Drug and Alcohol Abuse* 32:7–28, 2006.

Mumola, C.J. and Karberg, J.C. *Drug use and dependence, state and federal prisoners, 2004*. Washington, DC: U.S. Department of Justice, Office of Justice Programs, Bureau of Justice Statistics, 2006.

National Institute of Justice. *2000 Arrestee drug abuse monitoring: annual report* (pp. 135–136, Tables 6-2 and 6-3). Washington, DC: U.S. Department of Justice, Office of Justice Programs, 2003.

Office of National Drug Control Policy. *The economic costs of drug abuse in the United States,* 1992–2002. Washington, DC: Executive Office of the President, 2004.

Staton, M.; Leukefeld, C.; and Webster, J.M. Substance use, health, and mental health: problems and service utilization among incarcerated women. *International Journal of Offender Therapy and Comparative Criminology* 47(2):224–239, 2003.

Taxman, F.S.; Perdoni, M.L.; and Harrison, L.D. Drug treatment services for adult offenders: the state of the state. *Journal of Substance Abuse Treatment* 32(3):239– 254, 2007.

Taxman, F.S.; Young, D.W.; Wiersema, B.; Rhodes, A.; and Mitchell, S. The National Criminal Justice Treatment Practices survey: multilevel survey methods and procedures. *Journal of Substance Abuse Treatment* 32(3):225–238, 2007.

Teplin, L.A.; Abram, K.M.; McClelland, G.M.; Dulcan, M.K.; and Mericle, A.A. Psychiatric disorders in youth in juvenile detention. *Archives of General Psychiatry* 59(12):1133–1143, 2002.

U.S. Department of Health and Human Services, Substance Abuse and Mental Health Services Administration. *Results from the 2005 national survey on drug use and health*. Rockville, MD: Office of Applied Studies, 2006.

Volkow, N.D.; Fowler, J.S.; Wang, G.J.; Hitzemann, R.; Logan, J.; Schlyer, D.; Dewey, S.; and Wolf, A.P. Decreased dopamine D2 receptor availability is associated with reduced frontal metabolism in cocaine abusers. *Synapse* 14:169–177, 1993.

Volkow, N.D.; Hitzemann, R.; Wang, G.J.; Fowler, J.S.; Wolf, A.P.; and Dewey, S.L. Long-term frontal brain metabolic changes in cocaine abusers. *Synapse* 11:184– 190, 1992.

Volkow. N.D. and Li, T.K. Drug addiction: the neurobiology of behavior gone awry. *Nature Reviews Neuroscience* 5:963–970, 2004.

FOR MORE INFORMATION

For more information about other research-based publications on drug abuse and addiction, visit NIDA's Web site at www.drugabuse.gov, or call the National Clearinghouse for Alcohol and Drug Information at 1-800–729–6686.

INDEX

F

G

H

N

O

P

Q

R

S

T